ESTABLISHING AIR MEDICAL PROGRAMS FOR THE NEXT GENERATION
Frameworks for both Developed and Developing Nations

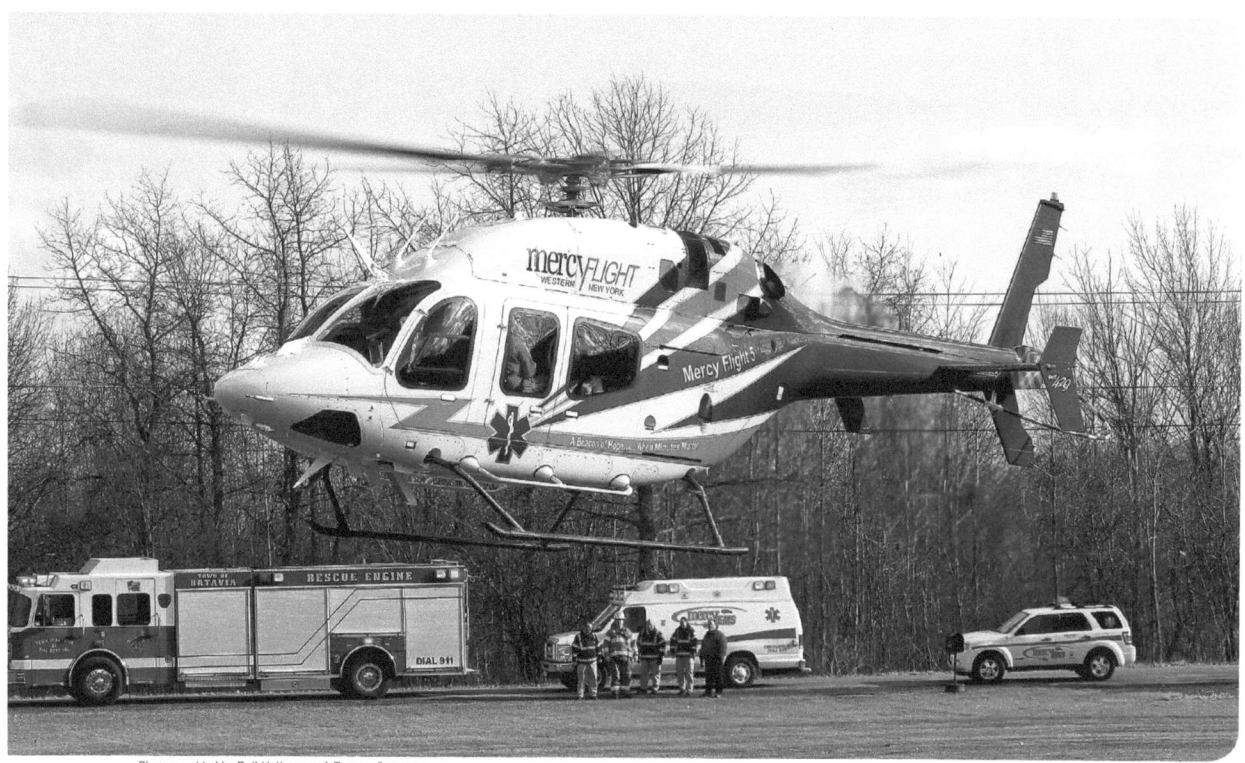

Photo provided by Bell Helicopter, A Textron Company

A project by the
Medevac Foundation International
www.medevacfoundation.org

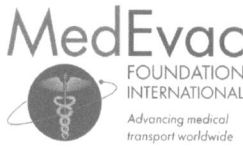

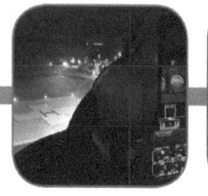 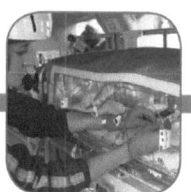 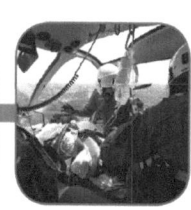

in conjunction with

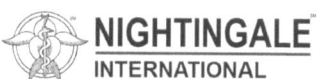

Funding provided by

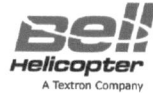

ESTABLISHING AIR MEDICAL PROGRAMS FOR THE NEXT GENERATION

FRAMEWORKS FOR BOTH DEVELOPED AND DEVELOPING NATIONS

A project by the Medevac Foundation International

www.medevacfoundation.org

Copyrght © 2017 Medevac Foundation International

All rights reserved.

ISBN: 1548465798
ISBN 13: 9781548465797
Library of Congress Control Number: 2017912821
CreateSpace Independent Publishing Platform
North Charleston, South Carolina

Table of Contents

	Introduction	xi
Chapter 1	Overview of Air Medical Services (AMS)	1
Chapter 2	Telemedicine & Onboard Internet Connectivity	4
Chapter 3	Planning or Auditing an Air Medical Program	9
Chapter 4	The Medical Component	17
Chapter 5	The Aviation Component	23
Chapter 6	Creating a Safety Culture	30
Chapter 7	Business Models for Air Medical Programs	38
Chapter 8	Air Medical Operations	43
Chapter 9	Air Medical Program Administration	66
Chapter 10	Air Medical Program Accreditation	73
Chapter 11	Air Medical Education and Training Programs	76
	Appendix A Civilian Aviation Administrations by Region & Country	81
	Appendix B A Quantiative Approach: the Precede-Proceed Logic Model	97
	References	109

Outline

Introduction xi

Chapter 1   Overview of Air Medical Services (AMS) 1
       1.1 AMS Policy Papers - Backgrounders 1
       1.2 AMS Brings Advanced Medical Care Directly to the Patient 2
       1.3 AMS Bridges Time and Distance, Flying Over the Barriers to Care 2
       1.4 AMS Extends Medical Care Beyond the Limits of Fixed Facilities 2
       1.5 AMS Delivers Efficient and Cost-Effective Critical Care Medical Services ... 2
       1.6 AMS Reduces the Time to Critical, Medically Necessary Interventions ... 3
       1.7 AMS Can be Faster and Safer than Ground Transport 3
       1.8 AMS is a Vital Resource Responding to Natural & Man-Made Disasters ... 3

Chapter 2   Telemedicine & Onboard Internet Connectivity 4
       2.1 Enabling Technology – Recent Advancements 5
       2.2 Telemedicine Enables Scalability and Capacity 6
       2.3 An Internet-Enabled, Onboard Mobile Medical Office 8

Chapter 3   Planning or Auditing an Air Medical Program 9
       3.1 Introduction 9
       3.2 A *Passionate Champion* for the Program 10
       3.3 Program Growth Stages: Capacity vs Sophistication 10
       3.4 Recordkeeping and Compliance: Manual vs Software 13
       3.5 A Quantitative Approach: *The Precede-Proceed Logic Model* 13

Chapter 4   The Medical Component 17
       4.1 Introduction 17
       4.2 The Medical Crew 17
       4.3 Training and Skill Sets 17
       4.4 Staffing Models 18
       4.5 Specialty Medical Crews 18
       4.6 Examples from Around the World 20
       4.7 Medical Direction 21
       4.8 Regulatory Oversight of Medical Staff 22
       4.9 Special Skills: Search and Rescue, Hoist Operations 22

Chapter 5   The Aviation Component 23
       5.1 Government Authority under Part 135 Regulations 23
       5.2 Flight crew 24
       5.3 Pilot Training 24

	5.4 Aviation Infrastructure, Aircraft Selection	25
	5.5 Airframe Modifications for Air Medical Operations	28
	5.6 Helipads, Landing Zones, Airports, En Route Infrastructure	28
Chapter 6	Creating a Safety Culture	30
	6.1 Introduction	30
	6.2 Safety Management Systems (SMS)	30
	6.3 Safety Management Leadership Academy	31
	6.4 Crew Resource Management	31
	6.5 Weather Reporting, Navigational Infrastructure	32
	6.6 Predictive Flight Risk Analysis	33
	6.7 Landing Zones	33
	6.8 Water Landing Egress Training	34
	6.9 Aviation Safety Technology	35
	6.10 *Helicopter Shopping* – Pressure to Fly Unsafely	36
Chapter 7	Business Models for Air Medical Programs	38
	7.1 Insurance by Third Parties	38
	7.2 Government Funded	38
	7.3 Government Subsidized	39
	7.4 Charity-Based Funding	39
	7.5 Corporate Sponsorship	41
	7.6 Membership Programs	41
	7.7 Hybrid Examples – Multiple Funding Streams	42
Chapter 8	Air Medical Operations	43
	8.1 Dispatch and Transport Mission Flow	43
	8.2 Dispatch and Transport Coordination	47
	8.3 Mission Profiles	48
	8.4 Bases and Operations Centers	50
	8.5 Infrastructure – Landing Zones	52
	8.6 Triage of Patients for Air Medical Transport	54
	8.7 Policy and Procedural Issues	57
	8.8 Operating in Military-Controlled or Conflict Zones	60
Chapter 9	Air Medical Program Administration	66
	9.1 Introduction	66
	9.2 Business Operations	66
	9.3 Staffing, Training & Human Resources	67
	9.4 Marketing and Public Relations	68
	9.5 Integration into the Local Healthcare System	69
	9.6 Medical Equipment and Medical Supplies	70
	9.7 Pharmaceuticals	70

	9.8 Laboratory ... 71
	9.9 Blood Products and Blood Banking ... 71
	9.10 Medical Records ... 71
	9.11 Cleanup, Waste Handling, Biohazard Disposal ... 71
Chapter 10	Air Medical Program Accreditation ... 73
	10.1 Program Evaluation ... 73
	10.2 Third Party Accredittion ... 73
	10.3 CAMTS - Commission on Accreditation of Medical Transport Systems ... 74
	10.4 NAAMTA - National Accreditation Alliance, Medical Transport Applications ... 75
	10.5 EURAMI - European Air Medical Institute ... 75
Chapter 11	Air Medical Education and Training Programs ... 76
	11.1 Medical Team Training ... 76
	11.2 Joint Medical and Flight Crew Training ... 77
	11.3 Training Facilities and Programs ... 77
	11.4 Full Mission Profile and Simulations ... 79
	11.5 Health Care System Training ... 79
	11.6 Professional Associations ... 80

Appendix A Civilian Aviation Administrations by Region & Country ... 81
Appendix B A Quantiative Approach: the Precede-Proceed Logic Model ... 97
References ... 109

Introduction

The Medevac Foundation International provides this guideline to establish, modify and sustain an effective air medical program. It serves as a resource for policymakers, regulatory agencies, and founding members seeking to establish air medical programs to serve their communities. This manuscript expands the description of air medical services to include a wide array of essential elements present in successful air medical programs. Throughout this document, we will present examples of successful air medical programs from around the world. And the following are some quotes from its air medical industry leaders:

"The Society of Aeromedicine Malaysia welcomes the landmark publication by the MedEvac Foundation International. We have been fortunate over the last five years from the time our Society was formed to benefit from the many interactions and learning opportunities provided to our members from our colleagues from all over the world. Being a service in its infancy, publications like this will help to further enhance our service delivery to be on par with the developed world standards. Without a doubt, the efforts of MedEvac Foundation International will be felt by patients in every part of the world who are at their most critically ill and requiring air medical services. Congratulations to the team for this valiant effort."

Dr. Gunalan Palari Arumugam, MBBS(UM), M.MED(ANES)(UKM)
Society of Aeromedicine Malaysia

"The MedEvac Foundation International is honored to have taken part in this extensive and exquisitely prepared landmark study designed to take the guesswork out of HEMS start up and also provides programs with a template to verify their current programs. While it contemplates the cultural, regulatory and country differences it establishes the basic safety, administrative and operational logistics for a well-integrated air ambulance service."

Johnny Delgado, MBA, BSM, EMT-P, CMTE, MTSP-C
MedEvac Foundation International; Chair, Board of Trustees

"This robust research project and publication, sponsored by Bell Helicopters and established by the MedEvac Foundation, strives to provide developing and developed countries with a framework to help deliver safe, effective and high quality based air ambulance critical care to patients and communities that

may not be adequately served. This work can be used immediately to help improve access to life-saving healthcare in countries or regions around the world."

David Evans, MA, ACP, CMTE
Association of Air Medical Services; Chair, Board of Directors

"This handbook represents a significant step forward in the advancement of air medical services. The methods put forward will help others establish and expand their services while the examples of next generation technology will help all of us continue to innovate and improve the services we provide. Congratulations to the Medevac Foundation for this accomplishment."

Christopher Manacci, DNP, ANCP-C
Chief Clinical Officer, Nightingale International LLC

"The Aeromedical Society of Australasia congratulates Medevac Foundation International on the compilation of such a comprehensive document, providing a "first template" guide for the development of a complete aeromedical service. Both new and existing operators in different parts of the world will benefit from the documentation of a framework based on wide experience and dedication to best practice. The clinical, aviation and managerial demands on even established organisations are becoming greater and more complex. This document highlights the need to ensure all elements of the business receive their due attention to manage these demands, while delivering a safe and effective service. It's an encouragement to all aeromedical organisations to see effort invested in a way that benefits the industry as a whole."

Mark Buick, BA Eng Aerospace
President, Aeromedical Society of Australasia

"The MedEvac Foundation, along with valued partner Bell Helicopter, recognized the need to educate any nation, currently without HEMS capability, on the unique and life-saving benefits provided by air medical services. HEMS programs undoubtedly benefit the patient population, but hospitals, businesses and local economies as well." said President/CEO for the Association of Air Medical Services and MedEvac Foundation, Richard Sherlock. The project, entitled Establishing Next Generation Air Medical Programs, is now complete and ready to be utilized to expand HEMS capability around the world in order to benefit of the world's most ill and injured patients."

Rick Sherlock, President & CEO
Association of Air Medical Services and the MedEvac Foundation International

"Helicopter EMS has become increasingly important in extending critical tertiary care to areas that would otherwise receive very basic care far from tertiary medical centers. As an increasing number of small rural hospitals close, HEMS assumes an even more important role to improve access to better medical care in *underserved areas. This document provides a thoughtful look at ways that HEMS can meet the challenges of future access to higher levels of medical care for a greater proportion of the population."*

Dr. Daniel Hankins, MD, FACEP
Emeritus Associate Professor and Consultant
Medical Director, Mayo Clinic Medical Transport
Past President, AAMS Board of Directors

ABOUT THE MEDEVAC FOUNDATION INTERNATIONAL

The MedEvac Foundation International is an international non-profit 501C (3) charitable organization headquartered in the Washington, DC area. The Foundation assists the Association of Air Medical Services (AAMS) to represent the Air Medical and the Critical Care Ground Transport Industry.

Since 2005, the Foundation has supported research, education, and outreach programs that enhance the industry's ability to provide quality medical care and provide safe and effective air and ground medical transportation for every patient in need. The Foundation funds programs and charitable activities that support AAMS' members and their families, who serve their communities with pride and commitment and provide life-saving services throughout the United States and around the world.

www.medevacfoundation.org

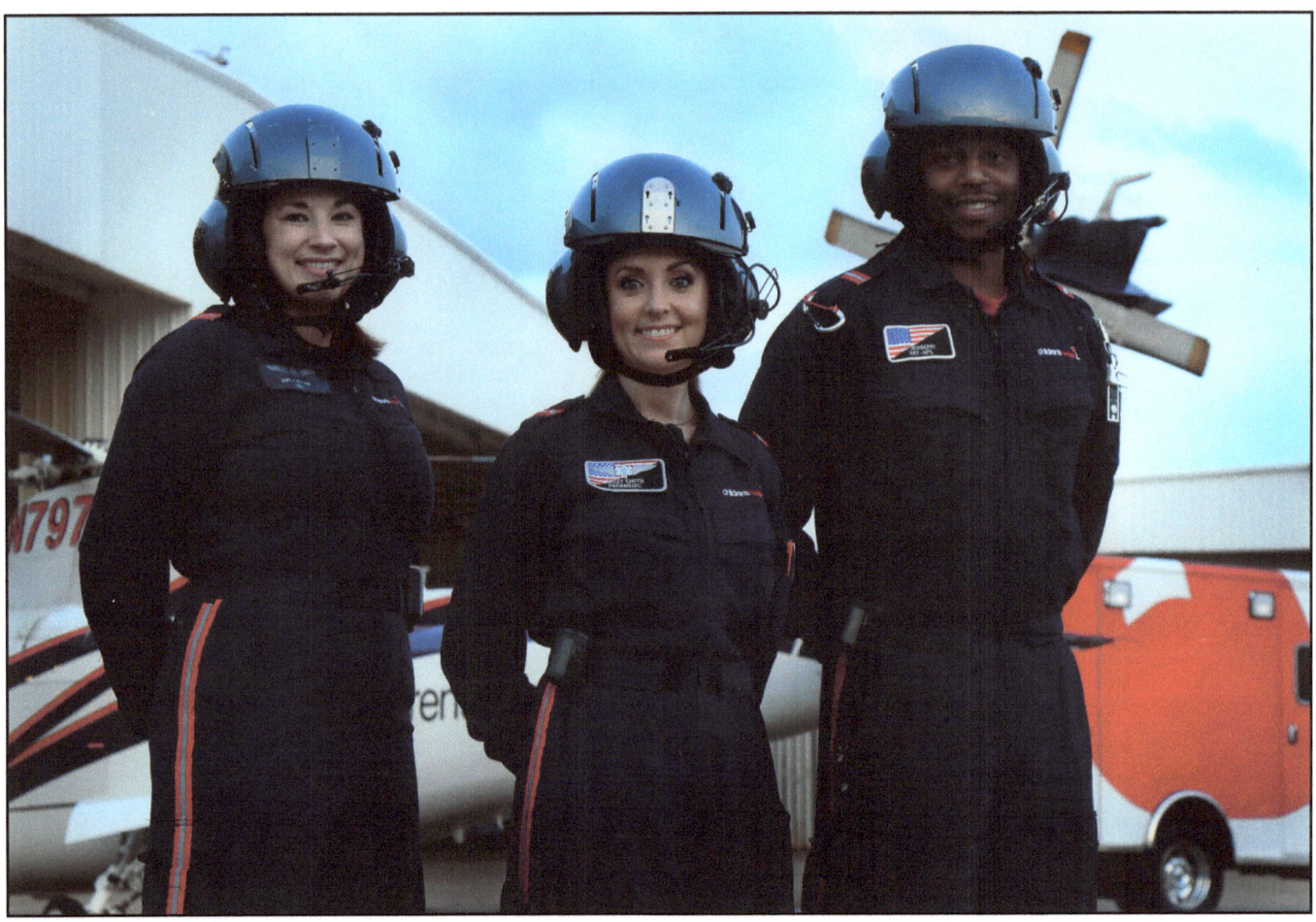

Photo courtesy of Mark Mennie Photography

ABOUT NIGHTINGALE INTERNATIONAL

Nightingale International (NGI) audits, plans, builds and maintains programs in emergency medicine, critical care transport, medical clinics and air medical programs worldwide. With its team of highly experienced industry leaders, Nightingale's programs improve patient survival and enhance clinical outcomes, as well as bring cost savings, increased control and more efficient resource utilization. NGI delivers integrated solutions to medical education & training, medical logistics, software implementation and integration, information systems, medical billing and reporting, communications and transportation management.

The group has extensive experience creating and sustaining both large and small scale programs in commercial, government and military sectors. Nightingale's team has significant operational experience in the U.S., Africa, Middle East, Asia, and other locations worldwide, especially in challenging environments.

www.ngi-med.com

CHAPTER 1

Overview of Air Medical Services (AMS)

1.1 AMS POLICY PAPERS - BACKGROUNDERS

Integrating air medicine into healthcare is essential at the local, state, regional, and national level. The recently published national consensus document, "Rural and Frontier Emergency Medical Systems Agenda for the Future," identified AMS as a vital component of rural and frontier EMS systems, and as the only Advanced Life Support-level service available in many areas of the globe.[1] It formally recommends that systems "plan, integrate and regulate, at the state level, aeromedical, critical care transport, and other statewide or region wide systems of specialty care and transportation."[2]

Air medical services saves lives and enhances access to critically needed medical care and rescue. As outlined in policy papers put forth by the Medevac Foundation, Air medical services are an essential element of contemporary emergency medical services. They revolutionize the ability of a medical system and its clinicians to reach critically ill patients and deliver life-saving care quickly and efficiently.[3,4]

In October 2009, the World Health Organization (WHO) convened a Global Forum on Trauma Care in Rio de Janeiro,[4] Brazil with a focus on international collaboration to improve access to appropriate trauma care globally and were composed of more than 100 trauma care leaders from 39 countries including physicians, Ministries of Health, Presidents of Associations/Societies (e.g. International Federation for Emergency Medicine, Network of Neuro-rehabilitation Hospitals, Bloomberg Family Foundation, the US Centers of Disease Control, and other health care professionals and society experts from around the world participated (full list of participants can be found listed in Appendix X).   According to the WHO, trauma causes 5.8 million deaths per year, over 90% of these are in low and middle-income countries. During the two-day meeting, participants reached consensus on a preliminary set of key messages to build a plan moving forward.

Every injured person should have:

- Basic lifesaving care in the field and rapid transport to a site of definitive care
- Access to adequate, timely, essential care that is life or limb saving at hospitals and clinics
- Access to adequate, essential rehabilitation services for those with disabilities resulting from their injuries.[5]

Establishing a new air medical program requires passion and determination aligned with a compelling purpose. Every air medical program in existence came about through the determined and persistent effort of passionate people working to solve the problem of getting critical care to patients in need. Today we stand on the shoulders of pioneers who combined their love of medicine and aviation to meet this critical need.

1.2 AMS BRINGS ADVANCED MEDICAL CARE DIRECTLY TO THE PATIENT

Air medical programs serve two purposes: to move advanced emergency and critical care to the patient and to move the patient to facilities of higher levels of care and recuperation rapidly. Optimizing both functions allows the most versatility and utility for air medical programs. Determining the best way to implement these goals requires a disciplined and organized approach.

Advancements in medical science, emergence of new technologies and the expansion of existing health systems drive innovation in air medical services. Where once it was considered enough to simply move a patient from the point of injury to a hospital, today's Helicopter Emergency Medical Service (HEMS) programs deploy highly skilled teams of highly trained clinicians armed with bedside laboratory equipment, ultrasound technology and invasive monitoring and life support equipment to the patient's location quickly and safely.[6,7]

1.3 AMS BRIDGES TIME AND DISTANCE, FLYING OVER THE BARRIERS TO CARE

Geography, terrain, and distance no longer dictate access to critical medical services.

Helicopters provide point to point transport and allow medical teams to access remote and unprepared areas. In heavily congested cities, air medical services can deliver a casualty to a hospital many times faster than a ground ambulance simply by flying over traffic congestion and terrain. For longer distances, fixed-wing aircraft provide timely access to care for patients in more rural or remote hospitals. Regionalization of tertiary and specialty care relies on air medicine to reduce the distance and time gap facing patients needing that level of care.[8]

1.4 AMS EXTENDS MEDICAL CARE BEYOND THE LIMITS OF FIXED FACILITIES

AMS has proven itself as an efficient and cost-effective way to expand access to emergency care and critical medical services, particularly in regions where the construction and maintenance of traditional brick and mortar hospitals proves difficult, illogical, or unsustainable.[8] Norway, the Czech Republic, and Australia, amongst others have successfully implemented air medical services to connect people in remote areas to centralized healthcare services.[9,10]

1.5 AMS DELIVERS EFFICIENT AND COST-EFFECTIVE CRITICAL CARE MEDICAL SERVICES

Critical care transport systems reduce time to critical interventions and make it possible for sick and injured patients to reach specialized medical resources quickly. These advantages result in healthcare system-wide enhancements in patient survival, reduced ICU utilization, and improved rates of recovery.[11,12,13,14]

1.6 AMS REDUCES THE TIME TO CRITICAL, MEDICALLY NECESSARY INTERVENTIONS

Critical care transport systems reduce time to medically necessary interventions and enhance access to specialized care resulting in an increased survival rate and reduction of disability from devastating injury or critical illness. Several papers demonstrate significant survival benefits for multiple injured trauma patients.[15, 16, 17]

1.7 AMS CAN BE FASTER AND SAFER THAN GROUND TRANSPORT

In many locations, air medical services can be faster and safer than ground transport for patients requiring timely access to critical medical service.[18-31]

In Buenos Aires, Argentina, traffic and congestion cause significant delays in the ability of ground ambulances to reach an ill or injured patient and bring them to a hospital. Fortunately, two distinct HEMS programs serve both the federal police service and the general population of Buenos Aires. Those HEMS programs fly with advanced practice (doctor/nurse) medical teams onboard and provide 24/7 service at no cost to the patient. They use small highly agile helicopters and frequently land on the city streets and highways in response to emergencies.

Patients injured or becoming seriously ill in foreign healthcare systems may require repatriation to receive the appropriate level of care and/or to avoid unnecessary economic and social costs from being away from their home country. Fixed-wing providers, commercial, or military aircraft play a role in permitting medical teams to safely transport such patients.

1.8 AMS IS A VITAL RESOURCE RESPONDING TO NATURAL & MAN-MADE DISASTERS

Air medical services also play a critical role in the response to natural and man-made disasters. Helicopters and their vertical lift capability are a highly versatile resource in support of relief efforts in both the civilian sector air medical programs and militaries across the globe. Judicious triage of patients and efficient dispatch of air medical teams can provide a critical lifesaving element in any disaster response.[32]

CHAPTER 2
Telemedicine & Onboard Internet Connectivity
The Next Generation of Air Medical Critical Care Systems

Air medical transport has become an extension of the hospital itself, providing critically ill and injured patients with state of the art acute medical and surgical care in a timely manner. Now, as Internet connectivity onboard aircraft and ground units is becoming increasngly available, it is possible to provide a much higher level of acute care diagnostics and definitive treatment during that first critical minutes of emergency response. Examples include portable MRI, portable CT scanning, and portable ultrasound for stroke patients; onboard portable laboratory analyzers and onboard robotic cameras enabling real-time consultation with critical care experts en route.

Internet-equipped air medical transport also enables the immediate retrieval of electronic patient medical records, diagnostic imagery, real time medical consultation, and insurance and other third-party payer information. In effect, the internet-equipped air medical service allows for near continuous contact with all involved parties throughout the transport, allowing greater team situation awareness, communication, and coordination.

Internet connectivity onboard aircraft has become increasingly available and affordable within the last few years, and now makes it possible to provide a much higher level of acute care diagnostics and treatment during that first critical hour of emergency response. Combined with the accelerating rate of development in telemedicine solutions, air medical transport is becoming an extention of the emergency room itself. This makes possible dramatic increases in favorable patient outcomes and more effective cost control – especially considering the downstream care given after the initial transport.

New medical diagnostic equipment solutions are continuously being developed, with smaller sizes, lower weights, increased data communications capabilities. Diagnostic tools such as ultrasound, x-ray, MRI or CT Scans are becoming more portable and lightweight. Further, the digitization of images and data are now allowing transmission to radiologists, receiving clinicians and other medical staff at other locations for preliminary interpretation. Emergency responders have better information within minutes as to how and where to transport the patient. Additionally, this diagnostic information can be immediately transmitted to the receiving care facility, giving them more time to prepare and allowing for prompt and more appropriate attention to the patient upon arrival at the hospital.

Today's portable monitors can connect to the internet and include several advances in mobilized diagnostic medical equipment such as integrated ultrasound devices, transcranial doppler ultrasound, impedence plethysmography, ETCO2, SvO2 monitoring along with traditional invasive line monitoring (arterial lines, pulmonary artery catheter monitoring, intracranial pressure monitoring), all of which can be transmitted in near real time via secure networks to remotely located experts for guidance, decision support, tracking, and record keeping.

2.1 ENABLING TECHNOLOGY – RECENT ADVANCEMENTS

Cost-effective, onboard internet connectivity systems have only started emerging recently. While analog communication systems have been a core component of most aircraft since the 1930's, digital voice and data communications have only been commercially available in the past two decades. Even so, it has only been since the last 4-5 years that cost-effective internet, Wi-Fi and voice-over-IP (VoIP) systems have existed for commercial and medical aviation use. Today, there are many new communications systems, hardware manufacturers, network service providers, and Part 145 avionics facilities that specialize in onboard internet and communications systems. Some of the major systems providers are Inmarsat, Iridium, Gogo, Viasat, Satcom Direct, Ligado, Thuraya, Honeywell, Garmin, Bendix King, and others.

Another long-standing challenge that has been resolved has been rotary-wing aircraft were previously unable to hold uninterrupted signal connectivity with satellite and other telecommunications due to signal disruption caused by the spinning rotor blades. As of mid 2016, new avionics and antennas specifically address this issue.

These new antennae and software upgrades synchronize with the rotor blades to communicate bi-directionally with the satellites using coordinated radio frequency bursts. This RF burst technology is currently providing up to 750 kps of bandwidth capability, and development is expected to increase.

To understand the layout of airborne cellular and internet connectivity today, the service coverages could be broken down into three categories:

1. Ground-Based Cellular Networks
2. Airspace Cellular (>10,000 feet, >3000 m)
3. Satellite ("Satcom")

All three of these service types enable both data and voice communications.

Ground-based mobile networks are primarily dedicated for mobile telecom, such as AT&T, Verizon, T-Mobile, Vodafone, and many others worldwide. Substantial infrastructure in these telecom networks has been built by both public and private enterprises. And in much of the developing world today, mobile telecom availability now reaches many of the rural regions in additional to urban centers. Aircraft while on the ground can connect to the internet and mobile telecom using the 4G, LTE, etc. with relatively high data speeds and lower costs.

"Airspace Cellular" telecoms leverage the existing ground-based networks by using the same ground-based cellular antenna towers, but focusing their reception and signals upward optimized for aircraft flying at altitude. As of 2016-2017, Airspace Cellular service has been available is most of North America and some parts of Europe, and new coverage areas are continually being developed in other regions. Through this type of service, higher altitude aircraft (i.e. airliners, private jets, etc.) have access to higher internet speeds at lower cost points than traditional Satcom connections.

Satellite-based communications are typically supported by either Inmarsat or the Iridium network of communications satellites. Coverage is mostly worldwide, but a few "dark spots" still exists where coverage is not reliable – mostly in some sparsely populated regions. Although these services offer relatively lower bandwidths and higher costs, the service is usually reliable whether on the ground or in the air, worldwide.

2.2 TELEMEDICINE ENABLES SCALABILITY AND CAPACITY

Analysts worldwide are projecting that the telemedicine market as a whole will more than double in the next five years (2016-2020). This exceptional growth will be driven by increasingly innovative telemedicine services and solutions, along with advances in the diagnostic and communications equipment to support them.

Some of the most significant segments of the telemedicine market are:

- Teleradiology
- Telecardiology
- Telepharmacy
- Telepathology
- Real-time video consulting
- Tele-ICU

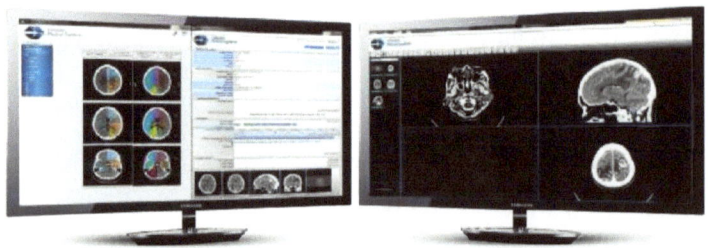

The general concept of telemedicine in the emergency response context is:

1. A doctor, nurse or other clinician performs diagnostic testing with a variety of medical equipment (portable ultrasound, portable x-ray, EKG, patient monitor, etc.).
2. That device takes the analog readings, and converts it into digital 0's and 1's, stored in local memory.
3. Then either this device will feed this data to its own screen or monitor, or it can transmit this same digital data out over the internet and to a remote screen or monitor, where a specialist can view and interpret it.
4. The interpreter then reports their interpretation back to the clinicians at the bedside, giving them the best information available from a reliable and experienced interpreter

Most major teleradiology systems communicate with each other, as their data imports and exports have been developed entirely DICOM compliant. One machine can accept a DICOM compliant images from any DICOM compliant imaging device. DICOM (Digital Imaging and Communications in Medicine) is the international standard for medical images and related information (ISO 12052), and defines the data formats and quality necessary for clinical use. DICOM standards are used in almost every teleradiology and medical imaging device worldwide.

Many innovative hospital and healthcare systems are starting to promote their new telemedicine capabilities as a key differentiator. Public police forces and government-administered emergency medical systems are adopting telemedicine initiatives to cut costs, while still increasing capacity and improving patient outcomes. Additionally, rural hospitals and clinics will have direct access to the internet to specialists, such as board-certified MD radiologists, cardiologists, neurologists, etc.

For example, each individual clinic usually could not afford a full-time radiologist on duty 24/7. However, they can contract with a company offering teleradiology services anywhere in the world 24/7, with 10-60 minutes turn-around-times (TAT).

The net benefit to an air medical program, and for that matter the emergency medical services program as a whole, is that telemedicine equipment, standardized data formats and internet-enabled aircraft, facilitate having a radiologist, cardiologist, and many other specialized medical service providers *virtually* onboard every flight.

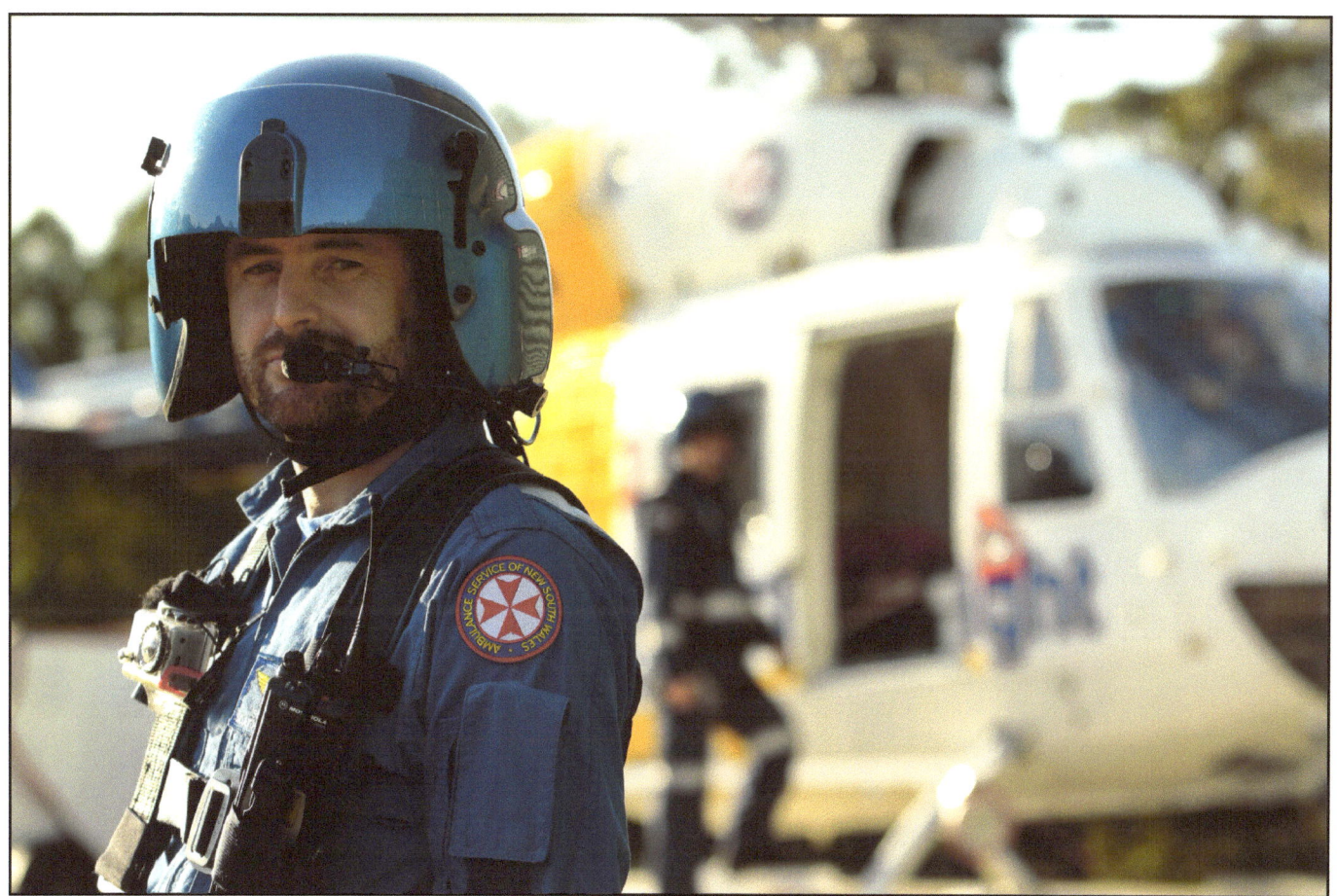

Photo courtesy of Mark Mennie Photography

2.3 AN INTERNET-ENABLED, ONBOARD MOBILE MEDICAL OFFICE

An internet-equipped, air medical aircraft can also serve as a mobile medical office while on emergency response missions. Ruggedized office equipment such as computers, printers, scanner and fax, are now available for installation in aircraft. This set of installed office administration devices make possible a wide variety of emergency medical tasks to be handled at the immediately and at point of patient contact.

Some examples of these time-sensitive, emergency response tasks are:

- Search and retrieval of medical procedure documentation
- Immediate retrieval of electronic patient medical records
- Diagnostic imagery and interpretation
- Real time medical consultation by specialists not onboard
- Insurance and other third-party payer information
- Sending and receiving of data files
- Barcode reader for administering pharmaceuticals and supplies

When planning out the flow and procedures of an air medical program, integrating this onboard mobile medical office into the emergency response process would enable better information communicated, sooner in the process, to improve patient outcomes, improve administrative control, and reduce costs – especially for the patient medical costs downstream.

CHAPTER 3

Planning or Auditing an Air Medical Program

3.1 INTRODUCTION

Air medical services expand the capacity and extend the capability of a medical system to deliver advanced care to people across a wider geographical area than traditional ground based emergency response systems. Successful programs meet a specific need in improving access to healthcare resources in a specific geographic region. The selection of the aircraft, the medical staffing model, and the medical services provided are typically chosen in response to regional needs, preferences, and available resources. Each program will reflect the preferences, culture, available resources, and level of investment by all stakeholders.

As you map out your program, here are some general areas of consideration:

- Medical Considerations
- Aviation Considerations
- Financial Considerations
- Creating a Safety Culture
- Business Models
- Operations; Workflow
- Program Administration
- Accreditation
- Initial and Ongoing Training

These areas overlap and significant interactions between them exist at all levels. Planning an air medical program requires a disciplined approach to the assessment of need and the careful integration of the two highly complex fields of medicine and aviation.

One approach we suggest involves the use a logic tool and process map in order to delineate as many variables and possible and create a useful assessment and plan. The PRECEDE-PROCEED logic model represents one commonly used logic tool for the assessment and planning of medical services that impact a specific population or health system deficit. We outline this tool later in this section.

3.2 A *PASSIONATE CHAMPION* FOR THE PROGRAM

Every air medical program requires a dedicated and passionate individual and/or group of individuals to carry out the planning and implementation of the program. These people are collectively referred to as Passionate Champions or Change Agents. Much has been written about creating organizational change with passionate champions.

This person or group of people would be the type that instinctively pushes for positive change in the program, despite the entrenched internal resistance to change common to most organizations. These people are willing to disrupt the status quo. They possess the strength, determination, and patience to endure the challenges associated with creating a new capacity or service. The passion they exhibit exceeds a simple emotional expression of support for change. Instead, they possess deeply held convictions that they express through commitment and hard work focused on the project.

In air medical programs, these individuals often come from the team of medical or aviation specialists involved in providing the service. More rarely there have been political or administrative personnel who provided the energy and determination to meet the myriad of challenges involved in setting up the program.

3.3 PROGRAM GROWTH STAGES: CAPACITY VS SOPHISTICATION

Setting up an air medical program may seem like a daunting task. While it does require significant sustained effort, each program results from a process and evolves through its response to challenges and opportunities to its current stage. Each program represents the cumulative efforts of the individuals and institutions involved, the sum of the outcomes of decisions and actions, and the various political, economic, and regulatory conditions impacting the program throughout its lifetime. There is no "one size fits all" blueprint. Each program grows in its own way and on its own timetable.

It may be tempting to think of development in air medical services in terms of the number of and types of aircraft used by the service or how many employees work for the service. While relevant to overall capacity and aviation capability, the absolute number of aircraft and staff does not in itself describe the true size and scope of a program. Just the same, describing the medical equipment or types of IV pumps and monitors does not adequately describe the service either. It will be easier to understand the growth and development of modern air medical programs by examining the program in terms of transport capacity and medical sophistication.

Transport Capacity

For this instance, we'll define *Transport Capacity* as the absolute maximum number of patients a program can serve in a given timeframe keeping in mind that serving a single patient per year requires the same infrastructure, number of staff and transportation assets as it takes to serve many more patients per year given the fact that one team using one aircraft can complete the first transport and be made ready to serve the next patient. Capacity also depends on the average trip duration, turn-around time, aviation variables, dispatch efficiency, alternative means of completing transports and financial considerations. It then follows that by increasing the infrastructure, staffing levels, transportation assets and operating efficiencies a program may be able to increase its capacity.

Medical Sophistication

We'll define *Medical Sophistication* as the scope and intensity of medical diagnostic and therapeutic interventions an air medical program provides its patients both upon arrival at the roadside/bedside and en route to the receiving institution. An air medical program with low medical complexity has limited medical sophistication and provides minimal care at the bedside/roadside and en route while a high complexity program will provide a wide range of surgical, emergency, and critical care services whenever and wherever they encounter a patient in need. Keep in mind this classification is largely artificial since many programs provide a broad range of medical transport and medical care services. Modernized air medical programs dispatch medical transport teams and onboard transport assets based on the needs of the patient and a determination of the most efficient and economical manner in which to meet those needs.

TRANSPORT CAPACITY VS MEDICAL SOPHISTICATION MATRIX

TRANSPORT CAPACITY ▲		
	High Transport Capacity with Low Medical Sophistication Medical escorts using commercial aviation represents a high capacity air medical service with low sophistication. Stable patients with limited medical complexity are escorted and assisted on passenger jets.	**High Transport Capacity with High Medical Sophistication** A program with several aircraft including several helicopters and fixed wing airframes delivering a wide range of medical transport services…
	Low Transport Capacity with Low Medical Sophistication Many air medical programs begin at this level. The aircraft may be simple, capable of transporting a medical provider to the patient. The care may be limited in scope and there may be little more than basic monitoring and basic live support available to the patient.	**Low Transport Capacity with High Medical Sophistication** This might be the next evolution of a program. The care delivered to the patient now includes critical care services and may include the benefits of a fully internet connected aircraft with a complete array of medical and diagnostic tools.
	MEDICAL SOPHISTICATION ▶	

Cost Savings and Improved Patient Outcomes as your Program Evolves

Evolving your program with increased medical sophistication, and inter-connecting with hospitals and other acute care providers, enables faster and more accurate diagnostic and procedure information. Often this can happen in that *golden hour* after the trauma has occurred, with the benefits therein being obvious to emergency medical providers.

And since the relative costs of the more sophisticated, internet-enabled medical equipment has been decreasing recently, equipping emergency medical aircraft has become more feasible.

Further, since more focused care may be given to acute patients earlier in the process, substantial cost savings may be realized by financial stakeholders in all downstream medical care. Air medical programs operate within the context of the larger medical system. Improvements in patient survival and improved outcomes in a variety of conditions, managed by air medical programs, can lead to cost savings across health care systems.

Cost savings accrue more quickly through matching medical sophistication and transport capacity to the needs of the patients served by the system. As a program grows to match the demand for service, more patients will experience the enhanced survival and outcomes provided by timely application of appropriate medical care and movement toward the most appropriate medical facility. Improvements in survival, outcomes, and the associated decreased utilization of healthcare resources result in decreased healthcare costs.

Matching Resources to Needs

Expanding the capacity and sophistication of an air medical program in any area will succeed best when matched to the needs of the community and the economic realities of funding the program. It makes sense to add to a program's capacity and/or sophistication if there exists unmet demand for the service and the funding and/or revenue streams will provide the money to support it. In some cases, a program may take on debt to finance an expansion if the leadership believes that the long-term benefits of expansion will allow the program to repay its debt.

Many programs experience periods of growth that involve a process of optimizing the utilization of existing assets, sometimes reaching a point of diminishing returns before investing in additional airframes and the attendant staff. Once the additional staff and airframe become operational the unmet demand will be met and the program can adjust its internal processes to best balance the workload across the entire service. Balancing these factors carefully and matching all areas to the perceived need will allow smooth transitions into higher capacity functioning.

Non-Linear Growth

It should be noted that increasing capacity and sophistication requires a comprehensive assessment of the impact of any changes prior to acting since each change will have a unique impact on the program and a specific financial requirement. Not all changes are equal. For instance, adding staff and management support to optimize the use of existing transport assets requires less financial resources than adding additional transportation assets due the overall cost of the asset and the need to increase staffing and management resources to optimize the use of the asset. This dynamic creates a non-linear step-wise growth pattern.

Examples from the Past

The earliest air medical programs developed by adding the transportation of persons with medical needs to ongoing aviation transportation operations. The airframes lacked medical equipment and may have had only limited modifications to accommodate a person laying supine. The earliest programs possess variable capacity and very low medical sophistication

During the Korean Conflict military helicopters transported numerous combat casualties to aid stations while providing little to no medical care en route. This represents a program with high capacity with low medical complexity. As time progressed, the medical complexity of the care provided en route increased exponentially.

In East Africa, a pair of volunteer doctors used their own single engine airplanes to reach remote villages to provide clinics and perform surgeries. Initially they used their own airplanes to reach the patients. They expanded service steadily through the creation of a foundation called AMREF (The African Medical Relief and Education Foundation). Today AMREF supports numerous health and education programs throughout East Africa, and has spun off a modern air medical service to provide state of the art critical care and emergency response air medical services across the region. Further, their operation has the ability to move patients around the world on modern fixed-wing, medical configured airframes. AMREF's efforts now impact the lives of millions of Africans every day.

3.4 RECORDKEEPING AND COMPLIANCE: MANUAL VS SOFTWARE

A core requirement with all air medical programs is recordkeeping and compliance. A variety of cost-effective software systems are commercially available, each focusing on a different part of the process. As part of the planning stage of a new air medical program, or potentially upgrading an existing program, it is highly crucial to map out the work flow and data required for reporting, compliance, and billing purposes. Some examples are:

- Dispatch Tracking & Control
- Billing, Medical Claims
- Claim Denial Management
- Analytics and Reporting
- Flight Planning
- Pilot Logs, Crew Duty Logs
- Inventory Control
- Controlled Substances/Narcotics
- Asset Management

- Fleet Maintenance
- Check Sheets
- RFID Tagging and Tracking
- Patient Medical Records
- Clinical Charting
- Medical Activity Logs
- Form Letters for Disclosure
- Compliance Logs
- Back-Office Accounting

In recent years, software systems have evolved to cover all of these requirements, and have developed interfaces so they can exchange data with each other.

Alternatively, these processes can all be done manually – as was the case until the 1990's. However, governments, health care organizations and insurance companies are more and more requiring that these processes be automated.

3.5 A QUANTITATIVE APPROACH: *THE PRECEDE-PROCEED LOGIC MODEL*

The PRECEDE-PROCEED logic model [1,2] provides a framework for the formal assessment of need and the development of an organized plan to address the identified need. The tool can be used to organize the plan and optimize the efficiency of creating an air medical program or improving an existing program. The specific requirements identified in the models various phases will serve as the focal point for program creation and on-going improvement. The subsequent data collection and analysis will allow for the creation of a project map and action plan. By identifying the necessary discrete variables that influence the practicality and sustainability of the program allows the leadership to focus their development efforts efficiently and effectively.

The diagram below serves as a visual representation of the cognitive process. The model flows from right to left along the top of the diagram for the PRECEDE component and from left to right along the bottom of the diagram for the PROCEED component of the workflow map.

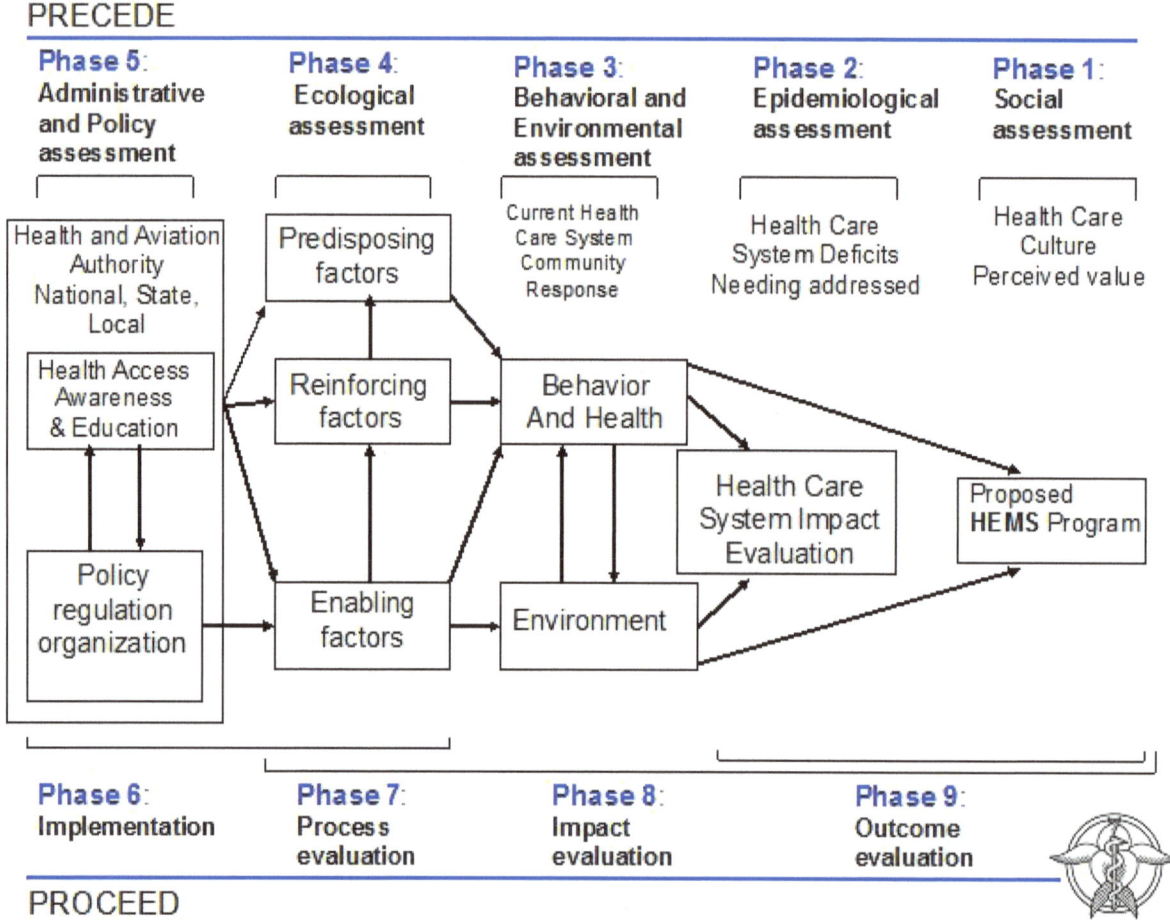

Addressing healthcare system needs requires the consideration of a multitude of factors and interrelated elements. Solutions to complex problems need not be complex themselves. Applying the method results in a highly organized data set and associated analysis which lends clarity to the development of an air medical program.

It is important that the mapping process and action plan possess three characteristics [1,2]:

- Fluidity: the steps in the planning process are sequential and build upon one another.
- Flexibility: the plan accounts for the needs of stakeholders and conditions that influence the proposed solution in ways that allow it to adjust to meet as many requirements as possible.
- Functionality: the plan results in an air medical program that solves the problem it was intended to solve.

The Precede-Proceed Logic Model is comprised of nine phases, or steps, as can be seen in the diagram on the previous page.

PRECEDE

The first component of the model is called PRECEDE which is an acronym for Predisposing, Reinforcing, and Enabling constructs in Ecological Diagnosis and Evaluation. This component captures all of the necessary objective and subjective elements in the existing healthcare delivery system and relates them to the requirements an air medical program will address. The first five sections organize the data collection and analysis according to discrete categories. As with any complex system, each factor interacts with each other factor. The Precede component allows identification of the myriad elements and the interactions between them.

    Phase 1. The Social Assessment:
    Phase 2. The Epidemiological Assessment
    Phase 3. The Behavioral and Environmental Assessment
    Phase 4. The Ecological Assessment
    Phase 5. The Administrative and Policy Assessment

Clarity comes from seeing the discreet elements individually and as they relate to each other and the whole. The linear organization of data and analysis helps identify what needs to occur before, during, and after in the planning process. Ultimately, the PRECEDE model helps organize data, and then analyzes and facilitates the creation of goals, action items, timelines, and budgets. When carried out correctly, each step of the process can be attempted in order, according to rank of importance and timing in the process.

PROCEED

The second component of the logic model is called PROCEED. This component includes the entire implementation and ongoing assessments of the air medical program. The last 4 phases organize the actions necessary to evaluate the impact of the air medical program and provides a framework to assess the impact of the program and ways it can be improved.

    Phase 6. Implementation
    Phase 7. Process Evaluation
    Phase 8. Impact Evaluation
    Phase 9. Outcome Evaluation

IMPLEMENTATION

The first five phases in the PRECEDE component involve considerable data collection and analysis and represent the entire body of information relevant to the creation of an air medical program. The accumulated analysis can then be used to guide all subsequent decisions related to the function of the program. While the logic model presents a linear process with discrete variables organized in orderly fashion the actual process will be dynamic. The implementation of the air medical program will require careful attention to timing, allocation of resources, and coordination of activities.

A detailed description of this methodology is included in the Appendix.

CHAPTER 4

The Medical Component

Successful AMS programs blend aviation and medical cultures into a single organization delivering safe, efficient, and effective high level medical and aviation services.

4.1 INTRODUCTION

The medical component of air medical services encompasses the entire range of equipment, expertise, systems and processes necessary to deliver lifesaving care using air transport.

Air medical transport places unique demands on medical providers and patients. Air medical teams often respond to the scene of accidents (Primary response) and other medical facilities (Secondary response) that possess limited resources. They must be able to work in resource limited environments while outside the hospital. At the same time, many patients they encounter require invasive procedures for stabilization and monitoring prior to and during transport.

4.2 THE MEDICAL CREW

Medical crews must account for changes in weather, moisture, and altitude to deliver the best care to a critically ill patient. Air medical teams face limits in the amount of equipment and supplies they can carry with them. Noise, vibration, and limited space create challenges in accessing and treating the patient during transport. Delivering care outside the hospital requires creative solutions and modifications to traditional procedures to allow air medical clinicians to provide excellent care in austere and chaotic environments.

Air medical crews often make use of ground ambulances as part of their work. They must be physically capable of lifting a patient, carrying bags of equipment, and climbing in and out of a variety of vehicles and small spaces. They must be familiar with the operations of the public safety, police, fire, and EMS services who call on them. Safety, leadership, and communications skills allow them to integrate into larger teams working at the scene of an accident or disaster.

4.3 TRAINING AND SKILL SETS

Most AMS programs provide new personnel with extensive training in air medical operations, safety procedures, aircraft familiarization, and competency evaluations by senior members. Initial staff members in a new program may benefit from spending time working with an established program to bring that experience to the new program. Increasing capacity and sophistication also requires formal training and implementing new management strategies and procedures. Formal education and training in air medical services greatly improves the efficiency of developing new air medical professionals and expanding the capacity and sophistication of existing programs. [1]

4.4 STAFFING MODELS

Air medical services requires motivated, energetic, professionals capable of working in challenging environments with unpredictable patient care scenarios. Most programs reflect the staffing patterns currently in use in ground EMS within the same area. The ideal team will consist of medical providers capable of correctly assessing and managing the patient to create the best outcome. Actual team compositions often reflect the local availability of medical providers, financial factors, and the local regulatory environment. AMS teams in Australia, Europe, New Zealand, South Africa and many parts of Southeast Asia often include physicians. Flight physicians typically have a wide scope of practice and their knowledge, training, and independent licensure allows them to triage patients on scene and perform invasive lifesaving procedures in the field. Independently licensed clinicians can also direct patients with less serious illness and injury to ground ambulances or even outpatient clinics where appropriate.

Each country regulates the practice and medicine and nursing differently, making direct comparisons difficult. Most flight physicians come from the ranks of anesthesiology, critical care, emergency medicine, surgery, and less commonly primary care. Many programs create specific programs to formally train their clinicians in air medical specific strategies and techniques.

The U.S. uses a variety of staffing models, including physician or nurse practitioner/nurse, nurse/nurse, nurse/paramedic, and paramedic/paramedic, nurse/respiratory therapist/EMT, and others. The change from physician-led medical crews to non-physician medical crews in the U.S. evolved as staff costs and third party reimbursement became predominant factors in program operations. Today, paramedics and nurses make up the majority of AMS medical crew in the U.S. The paramedic scope of practice tends to be narrower and well suited to primary (scene) patients where as a physician or delegated practice flight nurse tends to have greater scope of practice, more independent decision making capability, and skills useful for the care of secondary (inter-hospital) patients. Since most HEMS services are available for both primary and secondary patients, both skill sets are required.

4.5 SPECIALTY MEDICAL CREWS

Specialty crews often include providers qualified to provide care to patients with unique needs such as neonates, high risk obstetric patients, ventilator-dependent patients and those on life support systems and cardiopulmonary bypass. The configuration of such teams will be determined in each country dependent on local circumstances and is influenced by hospitals hosting such service and those on life support systems and cardiopulmonary bypass. In Australia, flight nurses often hold certification as a midwife which allows them to provide transport care to obstetric patients being flown in remote locations. Rega in Switzerland takes it one step further by utilizing rescue teams made up of physicians and paramedics at their high elevation locations. These teams are specially trained in rope rescue and high altitude operations. These teams provide advanced medical care to patients during rope rescue and long-line rescue operations and for those suffering from high altitude acclimatization emergencies.

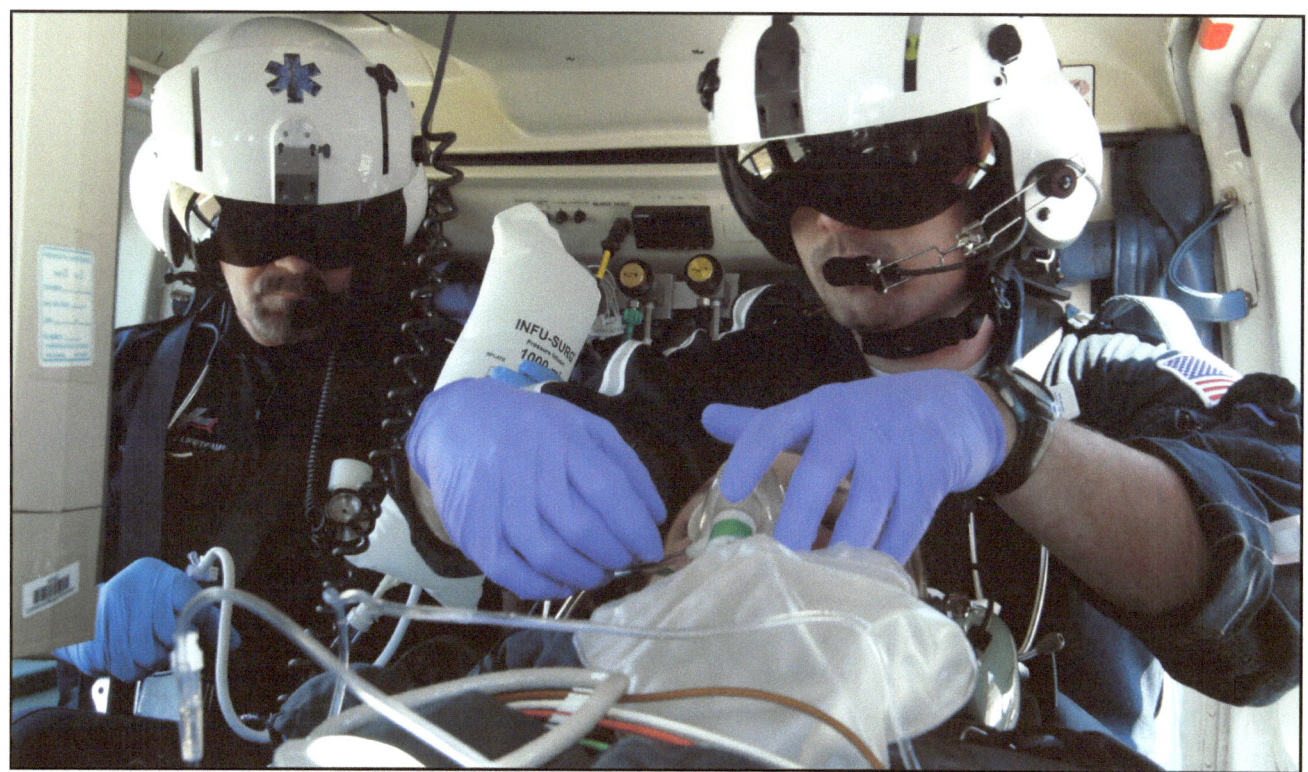

Photo courtesy of Mark Mennie Photography

Regardless of the clinical model, most programs use a minimum of two competent, medically trained, licensed/certified medical crewmembers during the transport phase of a mission. Ideally, at least one member of the air medical teams possesses the ability to perform the necessary invasive procedures to manage difficult airways and initiate invasive monitoring.

Several organizations are working toward the creation of standards focused on pre-hospital providers helping to ensure all air medical teams receive the appropriate level of training for operating safely in the aviation environment. Such standards are emerging through professional organizations including the Air Medical Physicians Association (AMPA), Air and Surface Transport Nurses Association (ASTNA), and the International Association of Flight Paramedics (IAFP).

All AMS medical teams must be trained appropriately for the challenging patient care they provide and operational environment in which they operate. They should be supported by appropriate continuing education programs and quality assurance processes X, Y. [2, 3, 4]

The medical crew should be comprised of highly trained professionals with extensive experience in emergency and critical care regardless of their title or professional credentials.

A full list of training topics and skill sets required for medical crew includes but is not limited to the following:

- Helicopter and fixed wing flight safety
- Emergency procedures in aircraft operations
- Water landing egress procedures
- Radio communications
- Accident scene operations
- Heli-borne search and rescue operations (if part of the service profile)
- Hoist operations (if part of the program service profile)
- Effects of air medical transport on patient care procedures
- Effects of temperature, moisture, altitude, and vibration on the patient and medical equipment
- Advanced medical and surgical skills for adult, obstetric, and pediatric patients

4.6 EXAMPLES FROM AROUND THE WORLD

Australia

Programs in Australia fly with physicians and paramedics (helicopter) and with physicians and flight nurses (fixed-wing). In some states physicians and paramedics are used in both fixed-wing and helicopters. In Australia, there is a distinction made between a "flight" nurse and a "retrieval" nurse. Flight nurses are required to also be a Registered Midwife, whereas retrieval nurses do not have this qualification. The rationale is related to the long transport times in extremely rural territories where local residents have limited, if any, access to birthing facilities and time-critical transport care of pregnant women is very common. Specialty programs for neonatal and pediatric transport generally use a doctor/nurse combination for all vehicle types. (NOTE: Flight nurses within Australia are predominantly used for fixed-wing transports.)

Czech Republic

In the Czech Republic, the flight physician usually possess specialization in emergency medicine, surgery, anesthesiology, intensive care, or pediatrics. They can also be a general practitioner but with special training in emergency medical procedures. Additional rescuers must hold at least a paramedic certification with a diploma-level qualification in EMS or a bachelor's degree, or be a registered nurse with a postgraduate specialization. Once again, all must be HEMS-Crew Members as detailed above following EU JAR-OPS 3 regulations.

Italy

In Italy, the AMS services fly with physicians, many with a specialization in anesthesiology. These medical teams include rescue personnel and other providers based on the geographic areas they service. High altitude bases often provide mountain rescue services while maritime districts may have experts in water rescue and hoist operations.

Japan

Japan recently expanded its air medical services coverage by implementing a university program training nurse practitioners to function as independently licensed providers on air medical teams. This required the country to create the nurse practitioner category within their national health system along with the requisite legislative modifications and educational programs.

South Africa

Programs in South Africa fly with physicians and paramedics having two years of experience as a minimum requirement, along with the traditional certifications of Advanced Cardiac Life Support (ACLS), Pediatric Advanced Life Support (PALS), Advanced Trauma Life Support (ATLS), etc.

Switzerland

The Swiss Air Rescue Service (Rega) utilizes the physician/paramedic team. Physicians work on a six-month contract and then return to their affiliated hospital. It is believed this system ensures the link between hospital and pre-hospital patient care management. Paramedics must hold a certificate from a college and fulfill European Aviation Safety Agency (EASA) flight crew licensing requirements and hold a HEMS crewmember certificate that is based on JAR-OPS 3 requirements. JAR-OPS 3 upholds a standard for training that includes completion of several layers of competency. The theoretical portion consists of 8 lesson units along with a practical part that can be completed in 2-5 days.

The team components include:

- HEMS-Crew Member as cockpit assistant
- HEMS-Crew Member as Paramedic
- HEMS-Crew Member as rescue operations expert

For details please visit: www.irs.eu.com/en/academy/specialisation-courses/hems-crew-member

4.7 MEDICAL DIRECTION

The AMS medical director provides essential medical leadership, oversight, and coordination of the medical service. They typically guide the development of routine and emergency care protocols, designate best practices, and participate in continuous quality improvement and research. The air medical service medical director can also be the liaison to local EMS agencies, hospitals, state and national professional organizations, and local, regional, and national partners. Several organizations exist to support air medical service medical directors including the Association of Air Medical Services (www.aams.org) the Air Medical Physicians Association (www.ampa.org)

4.8 REGULATORY OVERSIGHT OF MEDICAL STAFF

Most countries regulate the practice of medicine and nursing according to their requirements for professional medical care at an assured and monitored standard of quality and safety. There are historical, political, and economic realities determining which professional groups are involved in providing emergency response services, including air medical services. New programs must consider the scope of practice and availability of licensed providers when assembling flight medical teams.

Air medical operations also fall under the authority of the civilian aviation authority. Overlap between the medical and aviation regulations typically revolve around whether medical crews are recognized as flight crew and how medical equipment interfaces and attaches to the airframe. Air frame modifications for the installation medical equipment must meet stringent regulations. Further, flight crews must adhere to specific crew rest requirements. Medical team members are subject to the requirements of relevant work health and safety mandates under Occupational Health laws. There is a trend toward medical team members being subject to some or all of the civil aviation rules applying to flight crews as well. Air frame modifications for the installation medical equipment must meet stringent regulations. Medical equipment carried on board must meet safety standards mandated by the national civil aviation authorities.

New Zealand

New Zealand takes a national approach to the regulation of air medical services within its national laws. NZS 8156 sets standards of service for ambulance services including air medical. These standards include minimum requirements for medical staff credentialing and training. As stated on Verification New Zealand's website (www.verfication.co.nz/health/nzs-8156) "[NZS-8156] Provides a means of assessing the extent to which ambulance and paramedic services are worthy of patients' confidence and trust, through the demonstration of clinical safety, reliability, efficiencies, and effectiveness." The standard was introduced in 2002 and re-issued in 2008. The law outlines a certification process that includes a site visit for an audit to verify compliance. Additional surveillance audits are completed on an annual basis to ensure continued compliance and improvement. While New Zealand's smaller land mass and population may be seen to make developing such a countrywide standard easier, the development of standards are important to ensuring safe and effective AMS. There are a number of organizations who can help develop and implement standards in this area, including: the Commission on Accreditation of Ambulance Services (CAAS); the Commission on Accreditation of Medical Transport Systems (CAMTS); the National Accreditation Alliance Medical Transport Applications (NAAMTA); and the Association of Air Medical Services' (AAMS) Model State Guidelines.

4.9 SPECIAL SKILLS: SEARCH AND RESCUE, HOIST OPERATIONS

Search and rescue operations and hoist operations require additional specialized operational training and an intense cooperation between the rescuers on the ground, in the air, as well as the pilot in command. Any program that includes search and rescue work or hoist operations will benefit from the close advice and support of experienced search and rescue professionals.

In Australia, AMS helicopters are used routinely by the tasking authorities to undertake hoist and SAR mission.

CHAPTER 5

The Aviation Component

5.1 GOVERNMENT AUTHORITY UNDER PART 135 REGULATIONS

A core decision needed in starting an air medical program is how your operation will be authorized by your government to fly in that airspace. Generally, there are three categories of aircraft operating authority:

1. Civilian – Your government's civil aviation authority (CAA)
2. Military (military, coast guard, etc.)
3. Public Service (fire departments., police departments, forest service, etc.)

For our purposes, we will assume to operate under the CAA of your country. Each country has their own government civilian aviation agency (CAA), which has regulatory and oversight authority over commercial aviation activities. The following is an abbreviated sampling of some CAA's around the world; the entire list is included in the Appendix at the end of this book:

Afghanistan	MoTCA	Ministry of Transportation and Civil Aviation	www.motca.gov.af
Brasil	ANAC	National Civil Aviation Agency of Brazil	www.anac.gov.br
Canada	TCCA	Transport Canada Civil Aviation Directorate	www.tc.gc.ca
E.U.	EASA	European Aviation Safety Agency	www.easa.eu
China	CAAC	Civil Aviation Administration of China	www.caac.gov.cn
India	MoCA	Ministry of Civil Aviation	www.civilaviation.gov.in
South Africa	SACAA	South African Civil Aviation Authority	www.caa.co.za
U.S.	FAA	Federal Aviation Administration	www.faa.gov

Throughout the past three decades, the CAA's in almost all countries have standardized their aviation regulations to be mostly consistent from country to country. The regulations governing commercial aviation operations, including aircraft operating as air ambulances, are "Part 135" of those regulations.

The next step would be to decide whether to either:

a) operate the aviation part yourself, or
b) contract out to an existing Part 135 aircraft operator.

The requirements to maintain a Part 135 operation are extensive, but achievable. You will need substantial capital and time to build a Part 135 operation from the ground up. But this may be the best option for your air medical program, if you plan to start small with only 1 or 2 of the same type of aircraft. You can then scale up over time to a larger, more robust organization.

You should contact your country's CAA, and discuss their procedures, costs and estimated timeframes for building a new Part 135 organization. It would also be prudent to have discussions with existing Part 135 operators in your country, to determine if you could sub-contract the Part 135 part to them, and your group operates the air medical program as a whole.

5.2 FLIGHT CREW

Introducing helicopter services into an emergency response system requires a systematic approach and requires the involvement of competent pilots and aviation leadership. Each aircraft will be operated by a pilot in command (PIC). The PIC retains ultimate authority for all aviation operations and decisions to fly. Many programs operate with two pilots as part of their safety program.

The decision to operate with a single pilot versus adding a copilot depends on local factors and regulatory conditions. Safety data is highly variable on this topic with no conclusive studies to prove which option is safer. In Canada, the aviation authority requires two pilots at all times, day or night. The EASA requires a second pilot for night flying. In the United States, the majority of HEMS programs utilize a single pilot configuration.

The second person in the cockpit may not always be a pilot, especially for daytime operations. In this case, the second or non-flying person in the cockpit operates the radios, communicates with ground services, and acts as a second pair of eyes on the opposite side of the pilot during hoist/winch rescue work. Where larger or more complex fixed-wing aircraft and helicopters are used, the aircraft rather than the program may require a two-pilot configuration. For instance, most military and government run programs operate with two-pilot crews.

5.3 PILOT TRAINING

Aviation operations makes air medical transport unique among medical operational specialties. All aviation operations are regulated in many parts of the world but only minimum pilot experience and training requirements will be dictated by national general aviation guidelines. Pilot hiring requirements vary by program though most require minimum hours flying EMS missions. The majority of programs require their pilots to possess a total of 1,000 and 2,500 flight hours as pilot-in-command (PIC).

All pilots must be certified to operate the specific airframes used by the program and they must demonstrate competency in emergency procedures, navigation, and safe operation of the aircraft on a regular basis. Regular training and periodic re-certification is necessary for the pilots to maintain their skills and meet regulatory requirements.

The Aviation Component

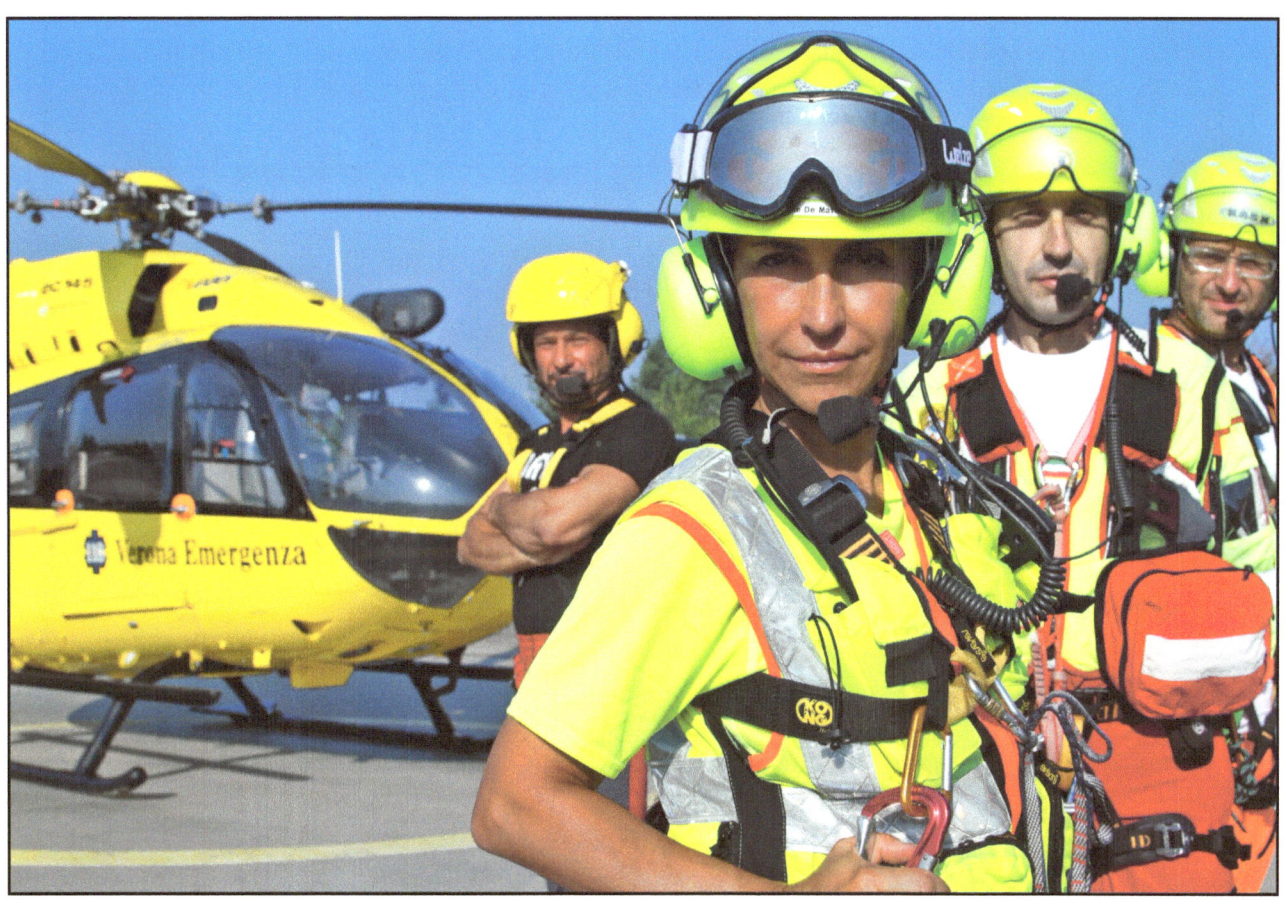

Photo courtesy of Mark Mennie Photography

In addition to the aviation regulator's requirement for proficiency and current training in normal and abnormal flight operations, IFR re-certification, AMS-specific examples include mission-specific training, crew resource management, integrating medical teams as an integral part of decision-making, night vision goggle use, hoist/winch operations, and safety culture training.

5.4 AVIATION INFRASTRUCTURE, AIRCRAFT SELECTION

Airframe Selection

Airframes selected for AMS must meet national, regional, and local authority specifications for patient transport and operational standards required for an aircraft-for-hire. If standard requirements do not exist, we recommend using the template outlined in documents available through the Association of Air Medical Services.

A wide variety of aircraft manufacturers and vendors provide an extensive range of models well suited to EMS. Choosing and integrating the helicopter or fixed-wing aircraft requires thoughtful consideration of the size of the geographic service area, its terrain, seasonal weather patterns, existing aviation infrastructure and the expected mission profile. Each airframe possesses different strengths in relation to suitability for specific environments, payload capacity, seating, interoperability, and operating costs.

It is imperative to look ahead and understand that the asset must fit your budget tomorrow. Maintenance and spare parts cost factor the biggest unless future budgets can assuredly meet future needs. Multi-use and diversification mitigate future cost challenges. Multi-use aircraft (EMS plus passenger / search & rescue) will, to some extent compromise your air EMS service quality. However, this may be worthwhile depending on circumstances - utility helicopters clearly suit multi-usage.

Another way to diversity that impacts future costs would be to create your own maintenance business and operation that could run as a profit center. At a minimum, this may bring down the cost of maintaining your aircraft(s) – especially if there are multiple aircrafts in your fleet. This also gives you control to ensure timely scheduled and unscheduled maintenance (*i.e.*, less helicopter "down time" due to maintenance). Further, this should ensure that you pay wholesale prices for spare parts and consumables. It is a risk to bring on the additional resources to run a maintenance, repair, overhaul (MRO) facility, especially if the MRO loses money. However, given that the biggest driver is maintenance costs (both labor and parts), your operation should be able to operate more cost-effectively in the long term.

Each airframe possesses different strengths in relation to suitability for specific environments. Here are some major factors and choices:

- Payload capacity
- Ceiling limit / power
- Seating
- Medical kits available or must they be customized
- Cabin volume and for EMS, the number of stretchers with equipment, medics available in asset
- Hoist capability
- Single or twin engine
- Single pilot or the addition of a copilot
- Decision to go with a different asset with different strengths or buy the same assets to keep spare parts, maintenance, pilot requirements the same with a consistent fleet
- Interoperability with existing assets or assets with other agencies
- Flexibility to do multiple use / tasks with the asset aside from AMS work; for example, search and rescue, passenger movements, cargo movements, sling load / external load usage – a utility helicopter with sufficient power is needed
- Availability of spare parts, especially if there are plans to operate in remote or austere environments
- In general, how long does it take to get spare parts and how proprietary are spare parts
- Cost of spare parts
- Regional familiarity with asset for pilots
- Cost and availability of training on asset
- Size of physical footprint - especially rotary wing diameter and length of fuselage plus main rotor reach in the front
- Cost of maintenance

- Calendar time expiration dates on major components, forcing overhauls after 5-7 years, even with low time flying
- Operational cost per hour
- Durability, especially how performance and "up-time" is impacted in austere places with dust, altitude, humidity, or extreme cold and heat
- Cost to buy new
- Relative cost of buying used or overhauled asset
- Cost of buying used or overhauled asset
- Cost of overhaul
- Relative resale value
- Is the selected asset certified by your local civil aviation authority (EASA in Europe, FAA in the USA, and typically CAA in most other countries)?
- Contract with an aviation company to provide "Part 135" aviation services and aircraft maintenance.
- Productivity-based contracts (Power By the Hour) options.

Some additional thoughts deserving consideration when selecting a helicopter for EMS Work:

- Single engine aircraft face operational limits when operating over open water and at higher altitudes.
- Used and overhauled aircraft can provide decent value for the money.
- Avionics are not proprietary to particular helicopters, and can be customized to suit the requirements for the types of work the aircraft will do - and your budget.
- Dust is one of the most troublesome aspects in austere environments.

In many instances air medical programs start within other utility or transportation services such as law enforcement, military, coast guard or search and rescue operations. They make use of the existing airframes in the parent program. The airframe configuration and performance capabilities are known. In this case, the service trains medical crews to integrate their activities into the ongoing mission.

For instance, the Federal Police of Argentina's Air Section in Buenos Aires, La Policía Federal Argentina (PFA), started with several multi-role airframes performing law enforcement support missions. They eventually found the volume of requests for air medical services grew sufficiently to justify adding additional dedicated AMS configured airframes. The choice of additional airframes was directly influenced by the program's industry relations and by pilot certification, maintenance requirements, and funding.

This determination should be made in concert with aviation and program experts within the air medical community to help ensure that the identified needs will be met. There is no one aircraft type or brand that can meet the need of every possible mission scenario. It is important to choose an airframe that will meet most of the current needs identified, have the fluidity to capture the potential for utility expansion, and can be supported in the region in which it will operate. The inclusion of specialty services and equipment such as cardiac assist devices, transport incubators, or biological containment units will also influence aircraft selection.

Decisions related to single engine versus multi-engine, single pilot versus dual pilot, visual flight rules versus instrument flight rules, and operational capabilities decisions are often based on existing national, regional, and local standards combined with the performance expectations. Local aviation experts, advisors from industry, and regulatory guidance will best assure the program selects the most appropriate airframe, avionics, piloting and contract support strategies.

5.5 AIRFRAME MODIFICATIONS FOR AIR MEDICAL OPERATIONS

Every airframe used in air medical services must meet the space and capacity requirements for patient care and staff needs. The airframe must possess the capabilities to carry and transport safely, the medical care team, the necessary equipment, and the patient (or patients) as appropriate for the expected range of operating conditions. This includes the fixed components of the air medical build-out, such as medical gas installations, power supplies, and communications systems.

All components should meet the spirit and letter of the regulations in respect to the safety of the patient exposed to the aviation environment as well as the safety of the medical and non-medical crew when exposed to the medical equipment in use. Preferably, system design should minimize variation in practice as a way of mitigating risks flowing from the variability of individuals working in the environment.

An example is having rigid methods of equipment and litter fixation rather than reliance on strapping methods which permit variation in practice. Certain modifications fall under the specific regulation of civil aviation authorities. Many manufacturers provide specific guidance in this area. Many aviation maintenance facilities possess the necessary expertise to guide new programs in ensuring compliance with the broad range of regulatory and safety issues related to air frame modifications.

5.6 HELIPADS, LANDING ZONES, AIRPORTS, EN ROUTE INFRASTRUCTURE

Landing facilities used by AMS should be appropriate for the expected scope of operations. In countries with poorly developed helipads and airports, hospitals and communities served by the AMS should be encouraged to upgrade to an extent which permits their maximum access to the benefits of the services provided. Examples include provision of hospital-based helipads with facilities for safe helicopter operations.

More distant communities served by fixed-wing may benefit from upgrading their airports to permit nighttime operations. Both may benefit from airways infrastructure permitting IFR routes, point-in-space GPS approaches, and night vision goggle procedures.

AMS operators are encouraged to advocate for such enhancements to the aviation infrastructure as a vital link in emergency medical care of critical importance to the communities involved.

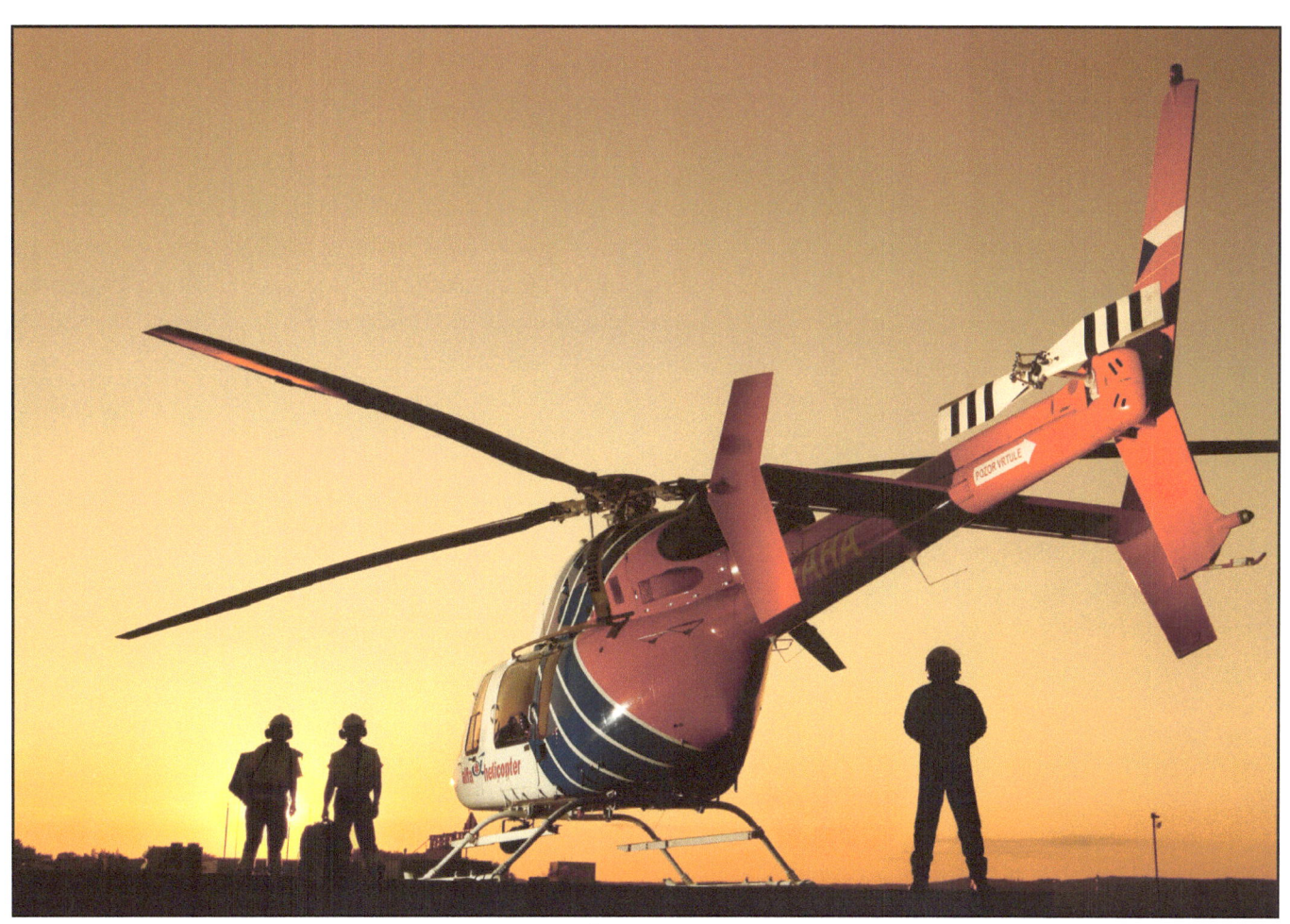
Photo courtesy of Mark Mennie Photography

CHAPTER 6

Creating a Safety Culture

6.1 INTRODUCTION

Air medical operations represent the combination of two highly complex industries. Air operations provide tremendous benefit to critically ill and injured patients and come with significant responsibilities for maintaining the highest safety standards and operational controls. The air medical industry developed a variety of programs aimed at creating a culture of safety within the industry. Today there exists a wide range of training programs, operating processes and systems available for integrating a safety culture into new and existing air medical programs.

6.2 SAFETY MANAGEMENT SYSTEMS (SMS)

In the U.S., the Federal Aviation Authority (FAA) defines SMS as the formal, top-down management approach to handling safety and risk, including the necessary organizational structures, accountability programs, and the requisite policies and procedures.

There are the four functional components of an SMS. These include:

- Safety policies which defines the leadership commitment to safety and includes methods, processes, and an organizational structure to achieve identified safety goals
- Safety risk management which includes the current risk mitigation controls in place
- Safety promotion which includes the training, communication and any other action needed to create a positive safety culture throughout an organization
- Safety assurance which evaluates the effectiveness of risk mitigation strategies in place and continuously assesses the potential for new risks

Formal training programs and online tools exist to assist in developing sound SMS within an air medical program:

- International Helicopter Safety Team (IHST) [1]: Formed in 2005, the IHST promotes safety and works to reduce civil helicopter accidents worldwide. The group's vision is an international civil helicopter community with zero accidents. IHST members work with various countries with significant helicopter operations to encourage accident analysis and the development of useful safety interventions. Partners include government and private participants from the US, Canada, Brazil, Japan, Australia, India, Russia, and

multiple countries in Europe, Central Asia, and the certain countries in the Middle East. The IHST offers multiple tool kits for small operators free for download: www.ihst.org.
- The Association of Air Medical Services (AAMS) introduced the Vision Zero initiative to decrease the accident rate through safety awareness.
- A Vision Zero[2] toolbox promotes the sharing of safety related practices with an online repository that is "filled" by industry experts and available as free downloads. (http://aams.org/vision-zero/)
- AAMS, in partnership with the International Board of Specialty Certification (IBSC), offers graduates of the Safety Management Leadership Academy the opportunity to sit for the Certified Medical Transportation Safety Professional (MTSP-C) specialty certification exam. The MTSP-C exam establishes a legally defensible and psychometrically sound examination that tests the science and application of the discipline of safety systems in both the air and ground medical transportation industry. The goal of the certification is to create an internationally recognized standard encompassing all aspects safety management and risk mitigation across the entire enterprise of medical transportation – with special emphasis on safety management systems, patient safety, and aviation/vehicle (aircraft or ground) operational safety. (http://aams.org/events/smta/)

6.3 SAFETY MANAGEMENT LEADERSHIP ACADEMY

In the United States, the Association of Air Medical Services (AAMS) introduced the Safety Management Leadership Academy (SMTA)[3] in June 2010 to meet a safety education gap. This is a two-year program delivered over one week each year. First year students cover topics such as accident causation/ investigation, SMS, human factors, regulatory considerations, balanced scorecard utilization, patient care safety, and more. Second year students cover additional topics including disaster management, safety culture, risk management, and take part in small group projects focused on scenarios such as post-crash incident planning, downsizing to smaller airframe, and many other topics. Additional information is available at www.aams.org.

6.4 CREW RESOURCE MANAGEMENT

Crew resource management (CRM) focuses on interpersonal communication, leadership, and decision-making in the cockpit. HEMS has the added component of a medical team and flight communicators (dispatchers) involved in every flight. Thus, CRM has been adapted to include all personnel involved in day-to-day operations. The European HEMS and Air Ambulance Committee (EHAC) is a trade association representing European organizations that provide emergency medical services by helicopter and fixed wing aircraft. In 2004, industry experts convened to develop Aeromedical Crew Resource Management (ACRM) which focuses on the human factor elements often attributed to accidents. Example topics include team-building processes, effective communication through development of a common language, changing the perspective between self-perception, and external perception. By utilizing reality-based case studies, participants immediately develop the relevance to their role in every day work experiences.

The Pilot in Command Must Have Sole Authority Over Aircraft Operations

The PIC has sole authority for the safe operation of the aircraft during every mission. Go/No go decisions should be made strictly on a flight planning assessment and flight conditions encountered once airborne. The medical scenario and demographics of the patient should not enter into the decision to attempt or continue a flight. Hoist or search or other rescue tactics should only be employed when there is no reasonable alternative and the PIC is confident that those operations can be conducted safely and within the regulations. Traditionally, the PIC remains blinded to the identity and clinical status of the patient to the greatest extent possible. This is thought to allow the PIC to make aviation decisions based solely on the appropriateness and safety of the flight conditions and aircraft status. All team members should work within a crew recourse management structure when communicating with each other. Medical crews should be mindful that the specifics of the patient's condition should not influence a pilot to make operational decisions. The specifics of the operational conditions should not influence medical decisions about a patient. For most patients there are alternative options as there are for most operational conditions, including the use of ground transportation.

Sterile Cockpit

The *Pilot-in-Command* ("PIC") controls the radio and only information immediately relevant to the operation of the aircraft is permitted. This generally applies in the startup, taxi, and departure phase and the final stages of approach and landing.

Initial and Recurrent Helicopter Simulator Training for Pilots and Crew.

All air medical programs must comply with local, regional, and national pilot training and recertification policies and procedures. The aviation industry also recommends initial and recurrent helicopter flight simulator training to establish and maintain proficiency in flight operations for expected scenarios encountered during routine operations, including the management of inflight emergencies and of inadvertent entry into instrument meteorological conditions (IIMC), a common challenge for helicopters operating in marginal weather conditions.

6.5 WEATHER REPORTING, NAVIGATIONAL INFRASTRUCTURE

All HEMS programs contend with variable weather conditions. U.S. programs benefit from a robust air navigation and weather reporting system. Pilots can rely on detailed and highly accurate weather forecasting and actual weather information in most parts of the country. In inclement weather, operating conditions can vary across very short distances. In many cases, weather information is not available for low-level operations or for landing zones and hospital helipads. Pilots may encounter adverse weather along the route and, if operating under visual flight rules (VFR), may have to abort the mission for safety concerns. They may be forced to land in a field to wait for clearing skies. Flying into clouds and becoming rapidly disoriented is an emergency situation called Inadvertent Instrument Metrologic Conditions (IIMC), and in too many cases this results in a crash causing loss of life.

As technology has improved, so has weather reporting capability, and the presentation of that information to pilots. While there is still room for improvement, some weather requires flight under instrument flight rules (IFR) and some weather conditions prevent flight at all but a few major airports. The risk of fog developing must be understood by pilots so they can make informed decisions about whether to accept or continue a flight.

Instrument Flight Rule (IFR) trained pilots operating IFR certified aircraft permit operations in weather known to prevent many types of VFR operations.

One method that some air medical operators have used was investing in the private development of Global Positioning System (GPS) based IFR procedures. These procedures can include precision navigational guidance for the en route, approach, and departure segments of a flight.

Programs in undeveloped regions must account for the lack of sophisticated weather reporting, en route IFR airways, approach and landing infrastructure. Whereas previously those facilities were highly expensive, modern technology is able to achieve equivalent and improved standards of aircraft operation with a move from ground-based aids to aircraft-based systems reducing the cost of greater reliance on the use of the IFR environment to conduct air medical operations.

6.6 PREDICTIVE FLIGHT RISK ANALYSIS

The decision to accept or decline a flight by helicopter typically involves evaluations of flight conditions such as forecast and actual weather and the availability of the IFR option in appropriate circumstances. Pre-hospital flights typically require visual flight, although in some countries this is no longer a requirement for the whole flight (e.g., Rega Swiss Air Rescue IFR to VFR). Recent developments in computer based decision support have led to creation of "go - no go" decision matrices. Helicopter flights can be analyzed for risk in advance by assigning numbers for dynamic and static elements, weighing each and then totaling up the score prior to a transport. Users can create a well-defined decision matrix for the pilot and team to use. There are numerous examples of flight risk analysis including some that are integrated into Computer Aided Dispatch software. One does not need to start from scratch to develop robust flight risk analysis. There are easily adaptable to programs unique requirements and should be a mandatory part of the pre-flight checklist. There has been less emphasis on advertising a specific launch time threshold as a competitive differentiator in the US. This is an effort to mitigate the pressure that could be put on a pilot to decide on inadequate information. The few minutes spent on performing a comprehensive pre-flight risk assessment pays dividends in patient and team safety.

6.7 LANDING ZONES

Designated Landing Zones (helipads)

Designated helicopter landing zones require extensive planning and investment. Access control and safety plans for the area around the helipad require detailed planning, documentation, and regular review and support. Costs are significantly greater for helipads installed on buildings or other structures. It is essential to work with experienced design and construction firms when installing or updating an existing helipad.

Helipads with anticipated high utilization should consider the inclusion of non-precision approach infrastructure to facilitate landings in an increased range of weather conditions, or alternatively, GPS approach and departure procedures.

Use an architectural or building firm with prior experience and understanding of requirements necessary to assure compliance with regulations (both national and local), insurance underwriters, and construction experts is essential.

Referring centers desiring to build a landing site to simplify helicopter operations and minimize delays in patient care should be advised on the correct construction and utilization parameters. Be sure to connect them to knowledgeable experts who understand the current and future requirements of helipad construction.

Emergency Temporary Landing Zones

Emergency temporary landing zones in urban, suburban, and rural areas present a unique situation for the pilot, flight crew, and ground personnel. All personnel must account for and manage numerous hazards prior to landing an aircraft in an unprepared area. Community-based emergency responders must be informed in the needs of a helicopter crew from ground personnel, the requirements for safely setting up an emergency landing zone, and the dangers associated with approaching the aircraft during emergency situations. Aviation experts and public safety personnel should be consulted to develop an appropriate outreach program for educating those who will be assisting in establishing landing zones on a regular basis. Most air medical programs sponsor landing zone education classes as part of their regular outreach to the community.

Pre-determined Temporary Landing Zones

It is often useful to establish pre-determined temporary landing zones in collaboration with local authorities. In densely populated areas, providers often designate landing zones to use as rendezvous points for ground EMS providers such as large parking lots, sports fields, and parks. Important additional information should also include obstacles and blade strike risks such as the presence of wires, trees, and other elevated hazards when choosing landing zones.

A great example of this type of collaboration can be found in Europe and Australia. Rega in Switzerland (www.helipad.com) and later Care Flight in New South Wales created web site www.helipad.org and began populating it with information about landing zones at hospitals, airports, military sites. They expanded their sites to include suppliers of fuel and much more including photos, current safety alerts, alternative landing sites, military installations, contact information, etc. Their sites gained traction with additional partners joining and adding even more information leading to a country-wide database with valuable information for any pilot.

6.8 WATER LANDING EGRESS TRAINING

A great example of a crew training innovation is the water egress training unit. Constructed using standard PVC pipe, this device is fitted with a seat and harness system and is pushed into a swimming pool while instructor-divers supervise the egress training of the helmeted and blindfolded students. Sophisticated versions (sometimes called Helicopter Underwater Escape Training) can include realistic helicopter interiors and some can simulate night time conditions.

6.9 AVIATION SAFETY TECHNOLOGY

The goal of this section is to highlight various tools, technology, and training that can help a program reach for the highest level possible in assuring a safe flight for the teams and patients. A list of available technological advances follows, though they may not be available and/or supported in every country. There are also limits on aircraft types that can support the technology.

The majority of aircraft crashes are caused by human factors. However, simply labeling the cause of a crash as "pilot error" offers no ability for others to learn from the incident. There are always several events that ultimately lead to an accident and identifying where such risk lies is key to any safety program. There is no "one size fits all" approach and thankfully many tools are available that can be customized to one aircraft or a fleet.

Global Positioning System (GPS) - is a space-based satellite navigation system that provides location and time information in all weather, anywhere on or near the Earth, where there is an unobstructed line of sight to four or more GPS satellites. Many programs in the U.S. have invested in remote GPS sites at referring hospitals, in addition to GPS mapped approaches to their primary receiving hospital in an effort to increase the ability to respond or adapt to inclement weather.

Wide Area Augmentation System (WAAS) – is a navigation aid to augment the GPS, with the goal of improving its accuracy, integrity, and availability. Essentially, WAAS is intended to enable aircraft to rely on GPS for all phases of flight, including precision approaches to any airport within its coverage area. Think of this as providing constantly updated safe lanes for aircraft identifying hazards such as terrain, obstacles, and other aircraft if also equipped with WAAS.

Helicopter Terrain Avoidance Warning System (H-TAWS) - aims to prevent "Controlled Flight into Terrain" (CFIT) accidents. The actual systems in current use are known as ground proximity warning system and enhanced GPWS and often these terms are used inter-changeably. The TAWS system has been in place for many years but geared mostly to fixed wing. This often causes false warnings since helicopters are flying at lower altitudes creating a situation where a pilot may disable the system to minimize the distraction. In recent years, H-TAWS has significantly reduced these false warnings.

Radar Altimeters – Radar altimeters measure the altitude of the aircraft above the ground (AGL) by calculating the time required to reflect radio signals transmitted from the aircraft. Knowing the AGL altitude of the aircraft can significantly increase the pilot's situational awareness and help to prevent controlled flight into terrain (CFIT) type accidents.

Aided Night Vision - Night Vision Goggles (NVG) have become a standard for programs flying at night in the U.S. and many other parts of the world. NVG's aid the wearer in seeing objects and terrain in significant darkness by amplifying dim objects thru technology that intensifies the original image into a much brighter scene. This technology can also be deployed by special night vision cameras which are typically fixed to the front of the aircraft but have the advantage of not requiring a NVG compatible cockpit. Those programs that fly at night have begun to acquire Night Vision Goggle experience and many programs are gradually putting their pilots through NVG training. Most offer in-house NVG initial and recurrent training designed with the typical EMS pilot in mind rather than accepting military NVG training.

Flight Data Monitoring Device - Flight operations quality assurance (FOQA)[4] utilized flight data monitoring devices placed in the cockpit to capture and analyze digital and in some cases photographic flight data generated during aircraft operations. The operator can use the data to identify and correct deficiencies during flight with the intent of reducing the risk of unsafe operations by offering corrective action in the form of training or counseling. This should be in a non-punitive manner (unless it was an intentional willful or repetitive violation) to build up the trust necessary in a strong culture of safety. (http://flightsafety.org/files/just_culture.pdf)

Aircraft *Health Utilization Management Systems* (HUMS) are systems which monitor engine parameters, vibrations, and other parameters that reflect the "health" of an aircraft and provide additional information to reduce aircraft component failure. These systems have been standard on larger aircraft in the oils and gas industry and are becoming more common place in HEMS aircraft adding an additional risk mitigation.

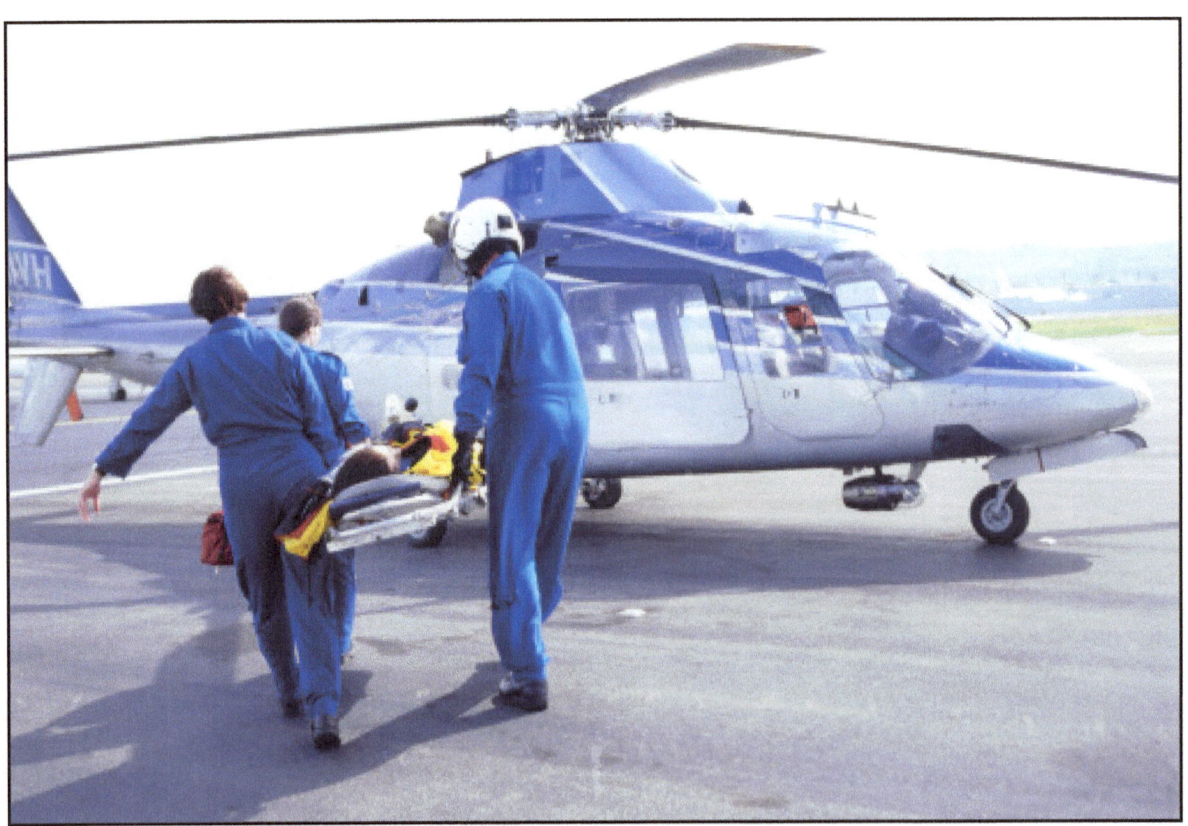

Photo courtesy of Mark Mennie Photography

6.10 *HELICOPTER SHOPPING* – PRESSURE TO FLY UNSAFELY

In regions where multiple services compete for work, a phenomenon known as "helicopter shopping" occurs. This phenomenon represents a tendency of referring parties searching for the most quickly available service to contact multiple providers simultaneously. The increased demand for service may create a situation where an air medical service may experience pressure to provide service under conditions that may be contrary to the safe operation of the service.

For example, some days may see every service in the region working to its fullest capacity. If requests for service outstrip capacity, it may create temporary shortage of available aircraft. When this occurs, services must triage calls for service and begin scheduling in advance. In response, referring clinicians and agencies may contact multiple AMS programs to find the program able to provide the fastest available response. During inclement weather, programs on the leading edge of a storm or weather system may determine they are unable to respond, where programs in areas the storm or weather system has passed, previously, may be able to respond safely.

All requests for air medical services must be evaluated and strict adherence to safety considerations (e.g., weather minimums, crew status, etc.) must occur at all times. Local and regional guidelines should require AMS programs to inform other AMS programs in their operating area when they have declined an air medical transport request. The sharing of that information will assist in mitigating a requestor from "shopping" for a helicopter or fixed-wing aircraft to complete a transport when they have already been informed that weather will not allow for safe flight. Further, programs should be required to educate requestors in their service areas on the dangers of "helicopter shopping."

CHAPTER 7

Business Models for Air Medical Programs

At the MedEvac Foundation International Global Forum held during AirMed 2011 in Brighton, UK, several business models were presented and discussed. The participants compared various strategies to determine which fundraising model best sustains air medical transport programs without compromising safety, quality, and innovation. Business models presented included:

1. Insurance by third parties (United States)
2. Government funded (Ontario, Canada)
3. Government subsidized (Czech Republic)
4. Charity-Based funding (United Kingdom)
5. Corporate sponsorship
6. Membership Programs
7. Hybrid blend of all of these funding methodologies (Switzerland)

Ideally, the cost of the service is spread amongst as many potential users as possible. Charging actual users alone places significant burdens on those users and discourages future use.

7.1 INSURANCE BY THIRD PARTIES

In the U.S. a large percentage of AMS providers collect the bulk of their revenue by billing the patient and the patient's healthcare insurance company. Patients without insurance are often billed directly.

7.2 GOVERNMENT FUNDED

In 1977, the Government of Ontario, Canada established a helicopter-based air ambulance program in association with Sunnybrook Health Sciences Centre in Toronto that included a training program for flight paramedics. It was initially called Ontario Air Ambulance. Since its inception the program continued to expand, adding aircraft and base locations. Within a few short years the organization became integral in connecting medical centers around the large province (~425,000 square miles) to the major medical centers in Toronto.

In 2006, Ontario Air Ambulance rebranded as "Ornge" Transport Medicine, and began functioning as a not-for-profit organization and a charitable foundation using a hybrid government-funded and charitable foundation business model. Ornge coordinates the air and land critical care, inter-facility transport system.

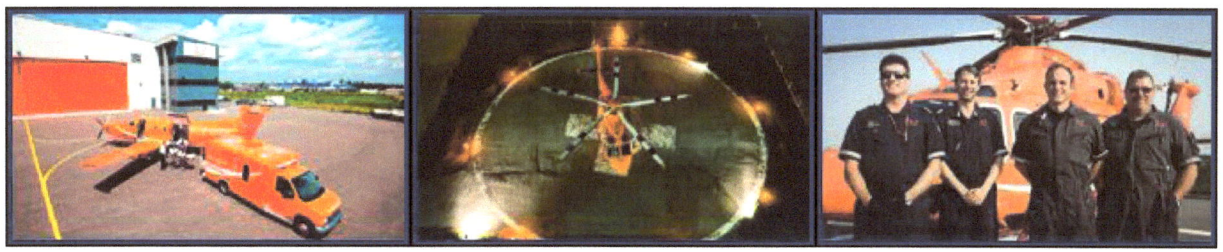

Source: Ornge, 5310 Explorer Drive, Mississauga, ON L4W 5H8, Canada, www.ornge.ca

7.3 GOVERNMENT SUBSIDIZED

In the Czech Republic, an interesting hybrid of funding exists. The Ministry of Health has undergone significant restructuring in recent years. They chose to rebuild the hospital based critical care infrastructure centrally and link outlying general care hospitals to these facilities using aircraft. This was seen as a more cost-effective solution compared to building multiple specialty care hospitals across the countryside. The Ministry funds the aviation operations while the medical program collects funds from the public health insurance program and the budgets of the regional governments where they are based.

The Czech Republic pays for readiness under contract (tender) and for variable (per patient) costs to appropriately compensate the providers. When a tender was released to provide air medical services for the country, the two existing private providers teamed up rather than compete to deliver a nationwide response network. They created mutually agreed upon service areas, clinical standards, pilot requirements, pricing, and aircraft requirements that were performance and capability defined, rather than of a specific model type of aircraft. This helped secure two Czech Republic based providers rather than an outside provider winning the 10-year contract. Having a long-term contract provides stabilization from both an economic and medical perspective that benefits the community and the government.

However, relying on government subsidy does mean the possibility of reimbursement variances should the country face austere times such as sometimes occurs in countries with commodity-based economies (e.g., oil, mining, agriculture, etc.). This also limits innovation (such as new safety technologies) because costs are not anticipated in the 8-10 year contract periods and typically must be pulled from net profits. It also limits the establishment of new transport programs when healthcare budgets are constrained.

7.4 CHARITY-BASED FUNDING

In some regions of the United Kingdom, air medical services are provided to its people through a charity funded service with each region having its own charitable trust. The charitable trust remains independent of the National Health Service and relies on donations from private individuals and corporations for operating capital. The providers prefer not to receive government funding from the National Health System (NHS), as it would entail NHS control of decision-making such as base location, utilization, aircraft model, and other areas of operation.

This has proven itself a successful albeit challenging business model as significant energy and resources must be spent in raising charitable funds. In any given geographic region there will be a limited number of large donors. Continuous fundraising efforts require significant manpower and time. Challenges arise when a significant donation has been collected from a donor by one region. The burden shifts from competing for patients, to competing for fundraising monies.

This model works well in places where the culture supports charitable giving and corporate social responsibility. Managing public perception of the value of the service takes many forms. Directly communicating to stakeholders in face to face meetings, written and electronic communications, sponsored fundraising events, and active participation with social media outlets are common strategies. In the UK a popular reality TV series called "Helicopter Heroes" messaged to the public a positive image of the value of air medical services. Episodes showed real life rescues of sick or injured people by helicopter medical teams. This is the kind of image where the message is "this could be me and I may someday need air medical services to rescue me", This makes an annual contribution to the local air ambulance trust an easy decision, but this image must be maintained and adverse public relations can be devastating.

Government Contracted - Charity Supported Air Medical Service

Many of the world's charitable AMS programs actively promote regular giving donations, and long-term business sponsorships, to provide them with sustainable funding. In some cases, the charitable service then contracts directly with the government to provide air medical services to discrete regions.

The Northern Territory of Australia possesses a massive land mass and a small population (230,000) distributed over a wide area. Few roads and challenging weather limits options for transportation, especially in an emergency. In response, the Australian government put out tenders for air medical services to connect the widely dispersed population to emergency care, midwifery support, and critical care transport.

The Australian Government awarded a contract to CareFlight (https://www.careflight.org.au/page/what-we-do/) based in Darwin. CareFlight provides rotor wing, Fixed Wing, personnel, medical oversight, coordination & dispatch and emergency response to an area encompassing the northern part of the territory. Additionally, the Royal Flying Doctor Service based in Alice Springs in the Southern part of the Northern Territory provides fixed wing service. Both services provide emergency response and midwife response to people living across a vast area that has very little healthcare related infrastructure. This program represents the first primarily air medical based emergency response system.

Non-critical transports by airplane are common, as are multi-patient transports to retrieve patients so that they can access centrally located facilities. For example, transports to psychiatric facilities that are uncommon in other parts of the world are common in the Northern Territories of Australia.

In the interim, the territorial Government closely monitors the service using Key Performance Parameters (KPP's). This territory had no benchmarks to start with so this is an evolving process. Triaging patients using strict medical controls has been a key part of keeping this service cost effective by shuttling lower acuity patients to higher volume multi-patient transports in fixed-wing aircraft.

7.5 CORPORATE SPONSORSHIP

Some air medical programs derive a portion of the necessary revenue to support operations from the generous contributions of large corporate entities. In some cases, these donations are discreet, in others, these donations are part of a deliberate and public display of support. In some cases, prominent businesses partner with communities to provide support for their air medical services. One such program in Buenos Aires, Argentina provides 24/7 coverage for the citizens of the city at no cost to the patients they transport. Public/private partnerships between governments, the communities and the businesses that serve them allow for businesses to demonstrate their commitment to the lives of their customers while also greatly enhancing the survival of those acutely sick or injured patients.

7.6 MEMBERSHIP PROGRAMS

A growing number of air medical programs of all types now sell memberships. The first membership programs covered fixed wing transports primarily. Membership programs initially began with an eye towards covering expenses for fixed wing transfers and repatriation flights. Today, several HEMS programs also offer membership programs. Memberships operate on the concept of collecting money from potential users to offset costs incurred by actual users and to pre-pay for flights they may need in the future.. In addition to simply collecting fees, the membership strategy also incorporates aggregate assessments and calculates the resources needed. Where aggregate risk is assessed, exposures are calculated, and resources are pooled. Rather than a charitable gift given without promise of returns, the membership represents a fee charged for specific access to the program.

The membership entitles the holder to access air medical service at either a reduced charge or no charge if a covered condition occurs. All memberships include a contract for service and terms outlining the specific services supported under the program. The members are typically recruited from the general population. The fee covers the costs of managing and marketing the program as well as the premium for an insurance policy covering the member.

There are a variety of options for organizing a membership program.   While there are a variety of ways to organize a membership program, most include some form of insurance. Two major types of insurance options exist for possible membership programs. The first, and more complex option, involves operating an independent off-shore captive insurance company. The captive insurance company must be formally established according to insurance regulations and possess cash reserves as required by law. The captive then writes performance contracts with the air medical service for its members. The performance contract covers the costs of service associated with covered conditions for service. In this way, the air medical service retains a potential user and has the reasonable expectation of having minimum costs covered should a claim for service arise. In the second, the insurance captive generates some revenue which they manage and from which they profit. Others purchase performance contracts from major insurance carriers for each member. The membership fee covers the costs of the membership program administration and to purchase a financial instrument that will cover the costs of a transport should the member request service under the membership contract. Typically, the membership provide members with the assurance of reliable and affordable service. The air medical program receives some revenue to offset the costs of maintaining 24/7/365 service.

7.7 HYBRID EXAMPLES – MULTIPLE FUNDING STREAMS

In Switzerland, Rega was started in 1952 to meet the needs of transporting patients in an extremely challenging geographical setting with high mountainous terrain and long ground transport times. Rega primarily relies on a donation program (formally known as a membership) from Swiss citizens, numbering 2.4 million patron cards issued, contributing SFr 86 million (USD $94m) in donations in 2011 alone. This is one method of spreading the cost to potential users of the service. This is in addition to insurance recovery when possible which is funded by actual users of the service. In 2011 Rega performed 14,240 missions with its fleet of 17 helicopters and three jets both in country and abroad (repatriation missions). It is important to note that the Rega service is available to every Swiss citizen regardless of whether they pay a donation or not, thus demonstrating how the hybrid model allows potential users to help fund actual users who cannot pay for these services.

In Alberta, Canada, the air medical service was started in 1985 operating under the auspices of the Lions Club, a registered charitable organization. The *Shock Trauma Air Rescue Service* (STARS) was incorporated in March 1986 as a registered charity and has operated as a hybrid model with minimal government funding, corporate sponsorship, and also charitable donations. Large fundraising efforts including the STARS lotteries bring in an annual revenue source over USD $90m, and include raffles of homes, vehicles, merchandise, etc. STARS Helicopters have corporate sponsorship names on them as well. This model has been very successful at linking community engagement, charitable giving, yet still charging the provincial governments for actual patient transports. STARS has expanded into the neighboring Provinces of Manitoba and Saskatchewan

CHAPTER 8

Air Medical Operations

8.1 DISPATCH AND TRANSPORT MISSION FLOW

Each patient transport starts with a request for service. The request may come from a hospital, a clinician in a clinic, a nurse tasked with arranging for a patient transport, a secretary in a medical unit, a family member, a broker, a public safety agency, or emergency responders caring for an injured person in the field. Regardless of who initiates the call, the request for service triggers several simultaneous processes.

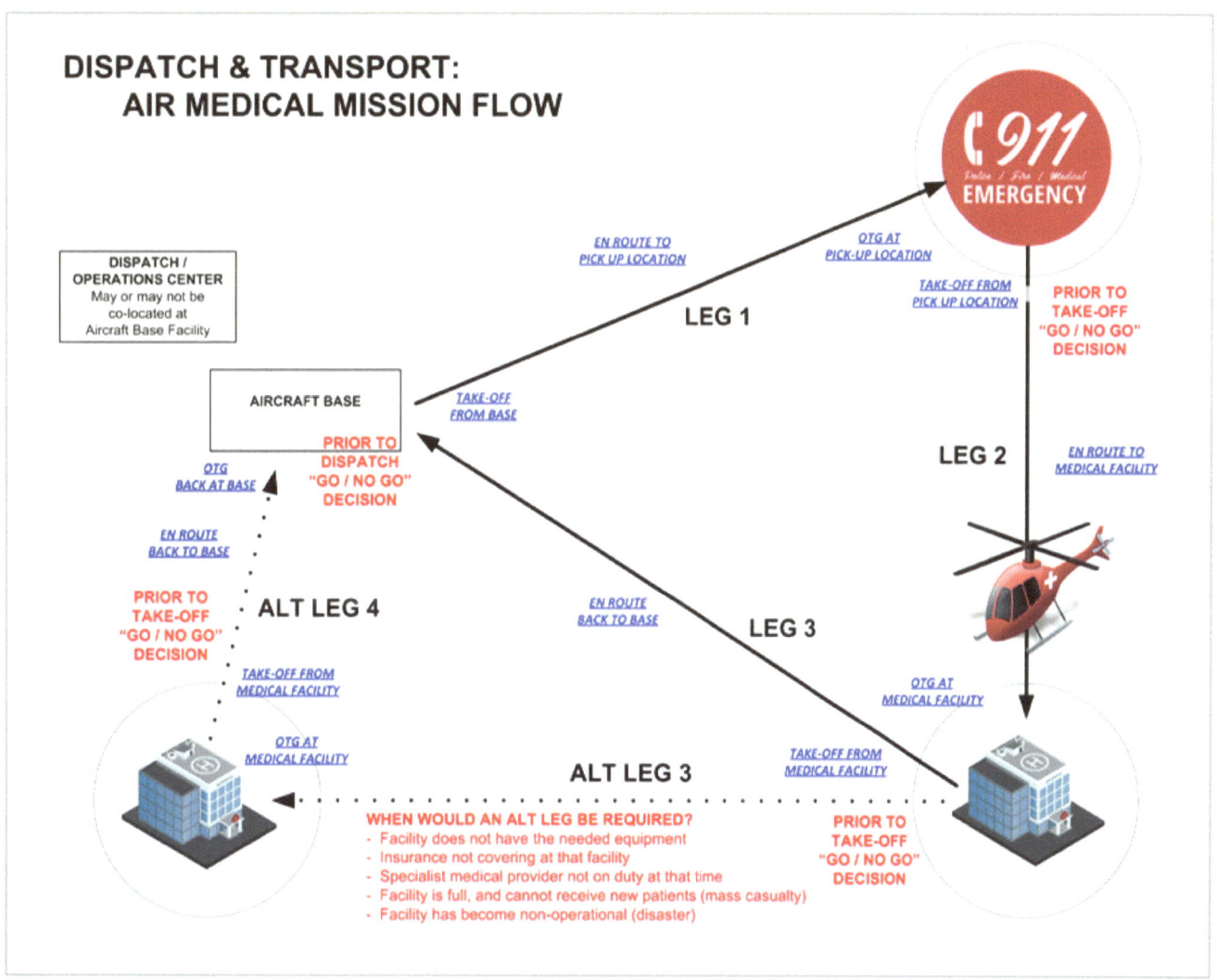

We'll discuss each process separately but assume that many of these activities will occur at the same time through the efforts of different staff within the air medical service.

1. Administrative Operations
2. Flight Operations
3. Medical Operations
4. Business Considerations

Administrative Operations

When a request for service comes into the program, whomever takes the initial call must attempt to gather as much specific information from the caller. The team will use the data to properly evaluate and respond to the request. A standard format of who, what, when, where, how and why questions will guide the requesting party to provide the required information.

The person taking the call represents the entire program to the requesting party and has the best opportunity to set the tone and pace of the interaction. Most programs develop a specific format or script used in answering requests for service and train their staff in the communication style best suited to maintain a positive working relationship with the requesting persons and efficiently gather the required information. Many air medical programs use specific forms or computer based dispatch software to document the time of the request along with the information gathered. In fact, some software programs allow for the creation of a complete transport record, including time stamps and entry fields for the flight risk analysis departure times, flight following and medical record.

All programs attempt to gather as much specific information as possible, including the patient's name, age, and medical condition. They attempt to gather detailed information about the patient's current location, the referring clinicians or agency, and specific contact information for the receiving clinicians, hospital and even a specific bed number or unit where the patient will go. In cases where the request comes from an emergency, the demographic information may be limited to gender and approximate age. The location information may be as simple as a certain highway mile marker, crossroads or GPS coordinates.

Additional information related to insurance coverage, payment for service and other financial considerations will reflect the business model and compensation methods in use by the service. Many of the financial and administrative functions will continue long after the patient transport has been completed.

The person taking the request then forwards the information to the air medical crews and other administrative personnel so they may begin to assess the request and plan the transport. Additional conversations typically follow, including discussions between the air medical program and personnel directly involved in the patient's care. This includes the clinicians involved in the transport request at both referring and receiving locations, patient representatives, regulatory agencies, business personnel and those responsible for arranging a landing zone and any ground transport for the patient and medical crew.

Flight Operations

As noted previously, the pilot in command bears the responsibility of determining whether a flight can begin or continue based on a formal flight risk assessment. It is important to allow the flight risk assessment to proceed quickly for several reasons. First, if a flight is not possible, the requesting party can be told to make other arrangements or the air medical program may continue to work with them to complete the patient transport when flying conditions improve. Second, the flight planning and coordination process requires time, time which is best used in moving the program into action and to minimize any delays of service. Lastly, the flight risk analysis will inform the medical crews about the conditions they may face during the transport and allow them to prepare in advance for them.

Once the pilot completes the flight risk assessment and has determined that a flight is possible, the flight crew begins planning the flight. The pilot must consider the weather along the entire route, the fuel requirements and refueling needs en route. The pilot(s) then make the airframe ready and prepare for the flight. As noted in previous chapters, most air medical programs prepare the aircraft for service immediately following the completion of the previous flight.

Once the transport has been approved, the pilot and any assistants develop the necessary plan to reach the patient. They may also file any required flight plans and obtain the necessary landing permissions with the civil aviation authority or locality as required.

Fixed wing transports often require formal flight planning and follow the standards set by the civil aviation authority for fixed wing operations. Fixed wing transports typically require medically appropriate ground transport from the airport to the hospital and back for the patient and medical crew in both the referring and receiving areas.

Medical Operations

As the pilot begins the flight operations process for the transport, the medical crew assesses the clinical and operational situation. It is critical that each transport plan account for the medical or surgical condition of the patient as well as precise information about the referral process and destination. The medical crew must prepare to interface with the medical staff and handle the logistical realities at both the referring and receiving locations, and they often consider other options for emergency care along the route should the weather or clinical status of the patient change in such a way as to require a deviation from the initial plan en route. The medical crew also determines if any special equipment or medications are required. Once they have a satisfactory understanding of the patient's needs and the operational conditions, they begin to prepare the aircraft's medical systems for the flight. Again, most programs prepare the aircraft for readiness immediately following the completion of a patient transport.

Business Considerations

Each request for service generates work for the program regardless of whether a patient transport occurs or not. Each program must determine its own business model and methods for revenue generation. It is beyond the scope of this chapter to determine how costs and fees are handled by the service.

Each transport requires the work of numerous staff along with the expense of maintaining and operating the aircraft and the medical equipment and supplies used in the care of the patient. In many cases, the transport records become financial documents used in accounting for the service provided to the patient. In fact, most programs document the various stages of the transport and create a medical record as part of the transport documentation. Many programs use specific software packages and billing technology to report the transport. Tracking these costs and submitting documentation and financial forms for reimbursement or budgeting requires additional time and energy. Programs often employ clerical workers and administrative or financial experts to assist the program in tracking costs and taking in the necessary funds to support continued operation. Alternatively, some programs have opted to outsource the tracking and billing function to third-parties that have specialized software and personnel to provide this service.

The Appendix section of this book provides examples of documentation, forms and references for specific software solutions used by some air medical programs to capture the pertinent information from the transport. – should we include specific examples of forms/recordkeeping/software?

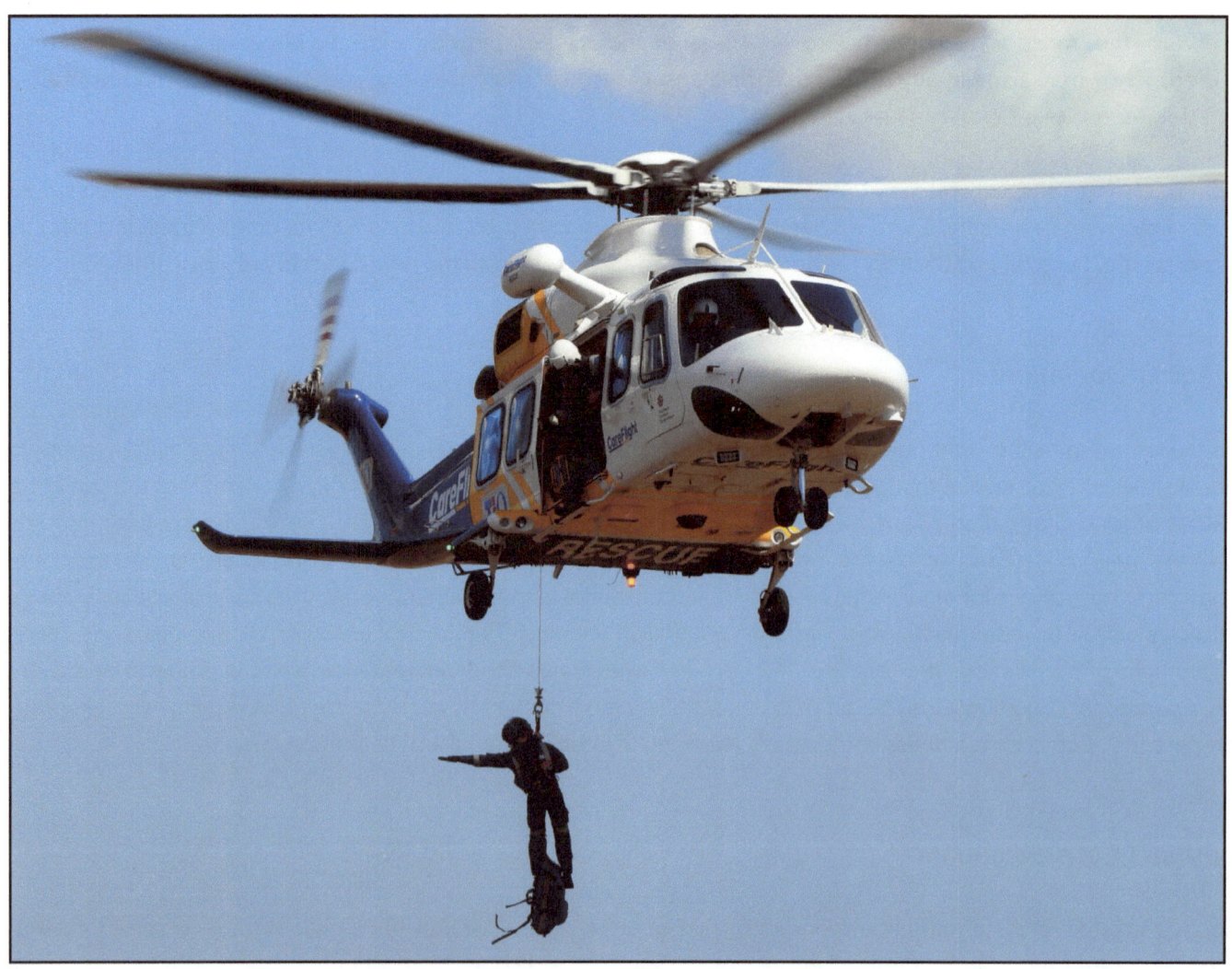

Photo courtesy of Mark Mennie Photography

8.2 DISPATCH AND TRANSPORT COORDINATION

Dispatchers and Communications Specialists

Each program requires the coordination of flight planning, medical planning and communication between all the various personnel involved in the care and transport of the patient. *Communications Specialists* perform this critical role, while leaving the flight planning aspects of the mission to the pilots.

On the other hand, *Flight Dispatchers* assist in the planning, coordination and monitoring of a flight, and may also coordinate communication between the other members of the service. In air medical services, they often have the dual role of communicating basic medical information to the medical crews. However, their primary responsibility lies with the flight itself.

Dispatchers require specific training and must be certified by the aviation authority of the region where they work. Depending on the governing aviation authority in the region, flight dispatchers may also possess the legal authority to alter, amend or cancel a flight plan depending on a variety of internal and external conditions. Prior experience with airlines and emergency medical services will greatly enhance the abilities of dispatchers to coordinate medical flights and emergency response coordination. While dispatchers may monitor other aircraft operating in the region, it is important to note that they are not a substitute for air traffic control in locations where they exist. . If AMS are operating under IFR plans, air traffic control has an obligation to monitor and control the flight; including functions such as aircraft separation that a Dispatch service would not normally provide.

Mission Coordination

The purpose of mission coordination is to assure a safe and efficient transport. Each transport reflects the unique aspects of the specific patient's needs, emergency situation and the complexities of clinical conditions a patient may experience. Coordinating the movement of a patient from one location to another by aircraft requires the assessment of many factors including location, flight planning, medical specialty information, acceptance at the receiving facility, availability of hospital beds and space, insurance or payment information, and finally, staffing and aviation safety considerations.

Flight Planning

Once the air medical service communicates with referring and receiving facilities and has confirmed acceptance of the patient the pilots can begin evaluating the safety of the flight and whether the crew can perform the mission. The dispatcher and pilots work together to determine the best flight plan according to aviation regulations, standards, and personal experience. Final acceptance of the mission and scheduling occurs once the pilots approve the flight and arranges for any navigational or administrative clearances required for taking off, flying and landing. If the mission requires an unprepared landing zone the parties responsible for meeting the aircraft will be apprised of their responsibility to assist the pilots from the ground to effect a safe landing. Preferably, the parties meeting the aircraft will have undergone landing zone safety training.

Medical Planning

Upon acceptance of the mission by the pilot in command, the medical team learns as much as they can about the needs of the patient prior to departure so they can assemble the necessary supplies and equipment and call in any specialist team members. In some programs, the senior medical team member participates in answering the initial call for service. This allows the medical team to gather as much relevant medical information as possible and assist the dispatcher or communications specialist with coordinating the hospital services in preparation for the patient's arrival. Most programs keep their aircraft fully stocked in anticipation of the next mission. Any specialized equipment or unique medications must be assembled prior to departure.

8.3 MISSION PROFILES

Each patient transport requires the combined effort of numerous individuals working alongside the medical and aviation crews to support and coordinate the air medical service. Every successful air medical program requires several dedicated, well-trained, passionate and talented people focused on bringing two highly complex fields of endeavor together to benefit people in need. The following mission profiles highlight the interactions of key program components alongside the variety of challenges faced by air medical programs operating in various roles and environments.

Primary versus Secondary Response

Air medical services provide a variety of response capabilities depending on the needs of their community and environments in which they operate. Most programs perform both primary response (contact with the patient occurs before they have been treated at a hospital) and secondary response (contact with the patient occurs after the patient has received hospital care). Both forms of patient contact require the same level of preparation and aside from differences in location and ongoing medical care, the medical crews must be prepared to manage any life-threatening conditions they find while continuing to support the ongoing care of the patient en route.

Below are some examples of various calls serviced by air medical services around the world. In each case the air medical service must demonstrate professionalism and expertise in a wide range of operational skills. All programs must plan for safety and efficiency during the transport.

Examples of Primary Responses

<u>Austere Environments</u> – Mountaineering accident involving an injured climber who has been initially treated by a wilderness medical provider on scene.

These responses usually involve ad hoc landing zones, minimal medical care prior to arrival of the team, and specialized skills to safely operate in a remote and hazardous environment. Hoist operations may require specially outfitted aircraft and specialized training for the crew and first responders. Medical providers must coordinate with other rescuers, pilots and receiving institutions to facilitate the best care for the patient. On scene and en route medical care will require providers to perform initial assessments and initiate resuscitation without the aid of hospital based diagnostic tools.

<u>Urban Environments</u> – Traffic accident involving a seriously injured trauma patient. The aircraft will have to land on the highway near the accident.

Air medical operations in urban environments require pilots and medical crew experienced in landing amongst buildings, overhead wires and urban infrastructure. Patients often require triage and stabilization by the medical crew and the team must work closely with first responders on scene to manage the landing zone, hazardous conditions and medical situations simultaneously.

<u>Suburban/Rural Environments</u> – Water submersion injury in a child who was swimming at a local pond.

Suburban and rural environments require careful attention to aircraft safety and efficient medical care. Like the urban scenario, suburban environments often include overhead hazards such as power lines, bridges and traffic. Air medical crews must coordinate with first responders to determine the best and safest way to reach the patient. In some cases, the air medical service can meet the patient at a predetermined landing zone near the scene after the patient has been moved by first responders. Examples of include playing fields, parking lots, or hospital helipads near the accident scene.

<u>Disaster Zones</u> – Crush injuries sustained by a pregnant female during a earthquake.

Disaster zones require air medical crews to expend additional effort to ensure the safety and security of the air medical team and patient. These environments often have limited resources to expend on assisting the air medical team in mission planning or execution. Disaster response must be coordinated with the agencies involved in responding to the situation. Air medical services should be considered a valuable resource that requires specific planning and careful utilization.

Communications and Ops Procedures

Once a request for a primary response comes in, it is essential for the air medical service to maintain contact with the agency/personnel making the request. Many programs utilize redundant methods of communication between the communications center, the aircraft, and the ground personnel on scene including cellular, satellite and radio communication when possible. Data collection focuses on pinpointing the exact location of the requesting party and the condition of the patient as well as any hazards present in the area. The air medical service may be required to give additional guidance to the referring party concerning the arrival of the aircraft and any delays that occur during the response. Basic instruction in marking the landing area may be provided as needed.

The flight operations for primary responses require careful consideration of the location and landing zone requirements of the aircraft. Most primary response transports begin with the aircraft landing at emergency and/or temporary ad hoc landing zones. This necessitates careful communication with the referring party concerning the arrival of the air medical aircraft. It may be necessary to coordinate with the referring party concerning management of any hazards in the area, and traffic control. It may be necessary to develop plans for the movement of the medical crew to the patient and the retrieval of the patient including the use of ground transport, or ropes and harnesses in the case of a fallen climber. Hoist operations require expertise on the part of the entire air medical team.

At the same time, medical information about the patient may be limited. The initial assessment of injury or illness may have been performed by non-medically trained personnel or by medical personnel with limited capability to treat life threats in the field. The air medical team may be the first medical providers on scene and must be prepared to initiate lifesaving therapy immediately upon arrival.

In many primary response situations, no formal attempt has been made on the part of the referring party to determine the destination of the patient, or whether the patient is able to pay for the service. Many air medical services arrange for the acceptance of the patient at a medical institution appropriate to the needs of that patient once the flight begins. Communication with the receiving facilities should begin as soon as reasonable. Many air medical programs have affiliations with their local supporting medical institutions to which they can make direct referrals.

Secondary Response

A secondary response transport typically involves moving a patient from one medical facility to another. As in the primary response, the medical team must be prepared to deliver a high level of care and provide emergency interventions. Examples of secondary response transports include:

Secondary response to a clinic or basic medical facility: A patient presents to a basic medical facility with a life-threatening condition which requires services and interventions in excess of the capability of the facility.

Secondary response to a hospital: A patient may require transport from one medical facility to another specialized facility capable of providing a higher level of care. Examples include trauma cases, stroke cases requiring neurovascular intervention and cardiac cases requiring cardiac procedures. The air medical crew must maintain the appropriate level of care en route.

Secondary response for repatriation: A patient may require transport from a medical facility in one country to a facility in another. In many cases, these transports involve the use of fixed wing aircraft and require additional administrative and flight planning time considering the need for medical visas, immigration and customs issues, navigation permits, the filing of flight plans, and coordinating staff to manage a trip that may take several days to complete.

8.4 BASES AND OPERATIONS CENTERS

Optimal service in HEMS includes a reasonable response time. Many programs base aircraft in locations that allow them to reach the patients quickly. This means they may have aircraft based away from the receiving hospital or sponsoring institution. Analytical tools can assist in determining optimum coverage areas and assist in determining the best locations for basing. [1,2]

The Communications & Operations Center

Called by various names, ("dispatch", "communication center", "transport operations center", etc.) and staffed by trained communications experts (dispatchers and/or communications specialists), these facilities form the hub of communication for the service. The communications center provides mission critical communication for medical crews and pilots to plan and support ongoing missions and assists in the coordination of business functions for patients, family members, doctors, emergency medical service personnel, insurance companies, other payers and other necessary parties.

The physical location of the communications/operations center varies based on the needs of the program. Many programs co-locate the communications center with the aviation program, usually at an airfield located in their service area. Some hospital-based programs operate communications centers out of the main hospital and stage aircraft at various locations within their service area to optimize response times. These programs use an airfield for maintenance and refueling purposes. Finally, some programs have separate locations for each major element of the service. The communications and operations center may be located in a convenient location apart from aircraft or hospital. The air medical teams and aircraft reside at strategic locations in the service area and the maintenance and inspection support operate out of a traditional airport nearby.

Under all circumstances, it is critical for the communications and operations center to develop and maintain excellent communications with the proper government (typically civilian) air traffic control authorities, especially at any airports nearby to ensure safety and proper coordination.

The technology used to communicate between parties involved in an air medical mission continues to evolve. In the past, a call for service typically came by telephone. Pagers and radios were used to communicate with medical crews and pilots. Today, most programs utilize several layers of technology to provide redundant and reliable communication between every member of the service and the referring and receiving partners. Technological advances in radio, cellular phone, internet and satellite communications hardware provide today's air medical programs with the ability to combine communications strategies into a variety of solutions. In addition, commercially available software systems allow users to capture patient medical and demographic data along with real-time communications, flight risk assessment, dispatch and flight following capabilities; allowing a program to record and manage every element the mission. These systems also create a record of the mission to use for business and continuous quality management purposes.

Transfer Centers

In recent years, many modern healthcare systems began integrating multiple aspects of their hospital admissions process, referral management and patient scheduling functions into unified systems. Healthcare institutions with dedicated air medical programs soon included their air medical communication, dispatch, and transfer coordination activities into that process resulting in what many programs now call a "transfer center". Transfer centers typically operate out of the main referral hospital in a geographical region. Referring clinicians and agencies can call one number and decide on the entire referral and transfer process, without having to make multiple calls to multiple distinct parties.

General activities of a transfer center include:

- Answer calls for service
- Facilitate communication between referring and receiving clinicians and accepting facilities
- Communicate with EMS, Fire, law enforcement, and internal healthcare facility participants to coordinate patient transport and emergency response
- Apply triage guidelines to coordinate multiple simultaneous requests for service
- Monitor radios, scanners, and weather channels for relevant information to ensure the aircraft is appropriately and safely dispatched
- Ensure the safety of the flight team by providing continuous flight tracking during patient transport missions
- Maintain communications with local, regional, and national air traffic control authorities
- Critical Incident management - Missing Aircraft Response
- Follow up with referring clinician/institution/agency for updates on patient status and feedback

8.5 INFRASTRUCTURE – LANDING ZONES

Designated helicopter landing zones require extensive planning and investment. Access control and safety plans for the area around the helipad require ongoing attention and support. Costs are significantly greater for helipads installed on buildings or other structures. It is essential to work with experienced design and construction firms when installing or updating an existing helipad.

Referring centers desiring to build a landing site to simplify helicopter operations and minimize delays in patient care should be advised on the correct construction and utilization parameters. Be sure to refer them to an architectural or building firm with prior experience and understanding of requirements necessary to assure compliance with regulations (both national and local), insurance underwriters and construction experts.

Unimproved and Ad Hoc Landing Zones

Impromptu or emergency landing zones in urban, suburban, and rural areas present a unique situation for the pilot, flight crew, and ground personnel. Numerous hazards must be accounted for and managed prior to landing an aircraft in an unprepared area. Community-based emergency responders must be informed in the needs of a helicopter crew from ground personnel, the requirements for safely setting up an emergency landing zone, and the dangers associated with approaching the aircraft during emergency situations. Aviation experts and public safety personnel should be consulted to develop an appropriate outreach program for educating those who will be assisting in establishing landing zones on a regular basis. Most air medical programs sponsor landing zone education classes as part of their regular outreach to the community.

It is often useful to establish pre-determined landing zones in collaboration with local authorities. Finding the most acceptable locations for landing a helicopter within their community. In densely populated areas not suited for ad hoc HEMS landing zones, providers often designate landing zone to use as rendezvous points for ground EMS providers such as large parking lots, sports fields, and parks. Important additional information should also include specific attention to obstacles and blade strike risks such as the presence of wires, trees, and other elevated hazards when choosing landing zones.

A great example of this type of collaboration can be found in Australia. CareFlight started a web site www.helipad.org and began populating it with information about landing zones at hospitals, airports, military sites. They expanded the site to include suppliers of fuel and much more including photos, current safety alerts, alternative landing sites, contact information, etc. The site gained traction with additional partners joining and adding even more information leading to a country-wide database with valuable information for any pilot.

In remote and austere environments, especially where dust is an issue, there are inexpensive solutions to creating cost-efficient landing zones using medium to large stones and "rhino-snot" / Envirotac to create an effective landing zone. Note that the stones must be large enough that the stones will not be moved by the rotary wing blades wake when the helicopter starts up, takes off, hovers and lands but not too large and uneven so that the helicopter cannot smoothly drive over.

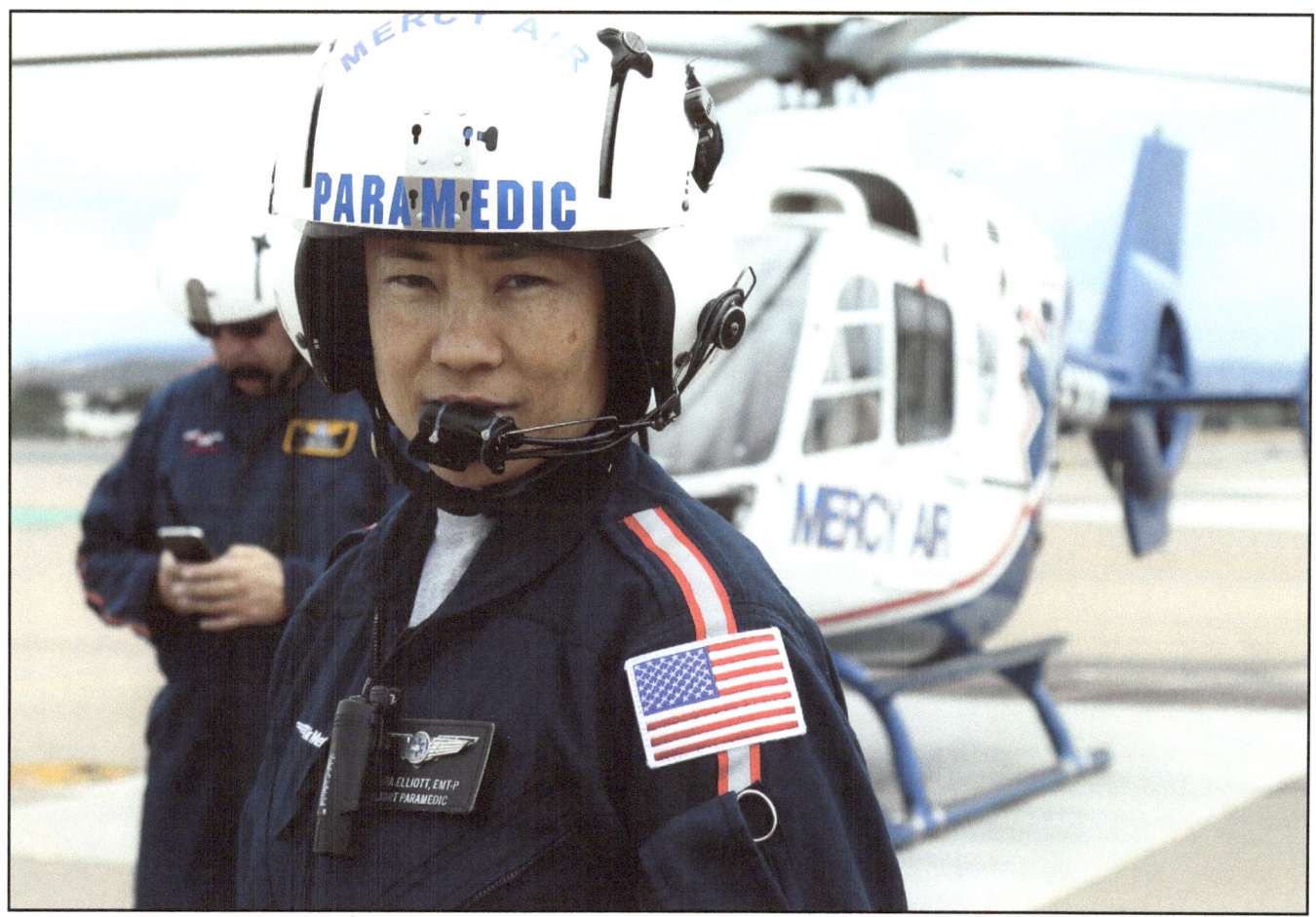

Photo courtesy of Mark Mennie Photography

8.6 TRIAGE OF PATIENTS FOR AIR MEDICAL TRANSPORT

In times of high demand, the air medical service may receive simultaneous calls for service that overload their ability to respond. In these cases, many programs use strict medical and operational criteria to triage requests for assistance and work to ensure that all requests are evaluated fully. In some cases, the programs schedule a lower acuity patient for transfer after responding to the more critically ill patients and emergency scenes. Patients with non-life-threatening conditions and normal vital signs may not require HEMS service unless other means of transport are unavailable.

Several authors [3-7] recommend developing specific clinical criteria to assist referring clinicians in determining the necessity of using the AMS service to facilitate a transfer. Recent studies show a rising utilization rate for AMS with a concurrent rise in the number of patients with non-life-threatening injuries.

Examples of Triage Criteria

Every modern healthcare system that includes helicopter air medical services must determine when to use the valuable and limited resources of the air medical service. Deciding which patients will best benefit from transport by air medical services represents a major challenge. Each program and their healthcare system faces the same challenge of balancing the need for matching patients to the best (life-saving and cost-effective) method of transport while minimizing the possibility of depriving a suitable patient with the best means of meeting their needs.

Many different triage approaches exist, many of which have been published online and are available for review. The following sets of criteria represent the most commonly cited examples. Many of the triage protocols focus on a disease process or category such as trauma, stroke, acute intracranial hemorrhage, aortic dissection. Other triage protocols focus on particular patients, such as obstetric, neonatal, or adult interfacility transports.

These tables that follow were cut and pasted from eb.medicine.net as possible examples of triage criteria which they have condensed from various state and national EMS association guidelines.

General Considerations

1. Patients requiring critical interventions should be provided those interventions in the most expeditious manner possible.
2. Patients who are stable should be transported in a manner that best addresses the needs of the patient balanced against the needs of the system.
3. Patients with critical injuries resulting in unstable vital signs require transport by the fastest available modality, and with a transport team with ant appropriate level of care capabilities, to a center capable of providing definitive care.
4. Patients with critical injuries should be transported by a team that provide intratransport critical care services.

Logistical Issues[8]

1. Access and time/distance factors
   a. Patients who are in topographically hard-to-reach areas may be best served by air transport
   b. In some cases, patients may be in terrain (e.g., mountainside, maritime, islands) not easily accessible by surface transport.
   c. Other cases may involve the need for transfer of patients for whom surface water transport is not appropriate from island environs.
   d. Patients in some areas may be accessible to ground vehicles, but transport distances are sufficiently long that air transport is preferable.
2. System Considerations
   a. In some EMS regions, the air medical crew is the only rapidly available asset that can bring a high level of training and capability to critically ill/injured patients. In these systems, there may be a lower threshold for air medical dispatch.
   b. Systems in which there is widespread advanced life support coverage, but where such coverage is sparse, may see an area left "uncovered" for extended periods, if its sole advanced life support assets are occupied providing an extended transport. Air medical dispatch may be the best means to provide patient care and simultaneously avoid depriving a geographic region of timely emergency response.
   c. Disaster and mass casualty incidents may make good use of air medical services.

Patient and Mechanism Issues

General Notes

1. In some cases (e.g., flail chest) the diagnosis can be clearly established in the prehospital setting; in other cases (e.g., cardiac injury suggested by injury mechanism and dysrhythmia) prehospital providers must use judgment and act on suspicion.
2. As a general rule, HEMS scene response is more likely to be useful when air transport results in more rapid patient arrival at an appropriate receiving center, or when helicopter dispatch affords rapid access to needed advanced prehospital care.

Scene air medical primary response is most likely to be of potential use in the following trauma situations:

1. General and mechanism considerations
   a. Trauma Score < 12
   b. Unstable vital signs (e.g., hypotension or tachypnea)
   c. Significant trauma in patients < 12 years old, > 55 years old, or pregnant patients
   d. Multisystem injuries (for example, long bone fractures in different extremities, injury to more than 2 body regions)
   e. Ejection from vehicle
   f. Pedestrian or cyclist struck by motor vehicle
   g. Death in same passenger compartment as patient

    h. Ground provider perception of significant damage to patient's passenger compartment
    i. Penetrating trauma to the abdomen, pelvis, chest, neck, or head
    j. Crush injury to the abdomen, chest, or head
    k. Fall from significant height
2. Neurologic considerations
    a. Glasgow Coma Scale score < 10
    b. Deteriorating mental status
    c. Skull fracture
    d. Neurologic presentation suggestive of spinal cord injury
    e. Acute changes such as stroke
3. Thoracic considerations
    a. Major chest wall injury (e.g., flail chest)
    b. Pneumothorax/hemothorax
    c. Suspected cardiac injury
4. Abdominal/pelvic considerations
    a. Significant abdominal pain after blunt trauma
    b. Presence of a "seatbelt" sign or other abdominal wall contusion
    c. Obvious rib fracture below the nipple line
    d. Major pelvic fracture (e.g., unstable pelvic ring disruption, open pelvic fracture, or pelvic fracture with hypotension)
5. Orthopedic/extremity considerations
    a. Partial or total amputation of a limb (exclusive of digits
    b. Finger/thumb amputation when emergent surgical evaluation (i.e., for replantation consideration) is indicated and rapid surface transport is not available
    c. Fracture or dislocation with vascular compromise
    d. Extremity ischemia
    e. Open long bone fractures
    f. Two or more long bone fractures
6. Major burns
    a. > 20% body surface area
    b. Involvement of face, head, hands, feet, or genitalia
    c. Inhalational injury
    d. Electrical or chemical burns
    e. Burns with associated injuries
    f. Patients with near drowning injuries

Questions that can Assist in Determining Appropriate Transport Mode [8,9]

- Does the patient's clinical condition require minimization of time spent out of the hospital environment during the transport?
- Does the patient require specific or time-sensitive evaluation or treatment that is not available at the referring facility?
- Is the patient located in an area that is inaccessible to ground transport?

- What are the current and predicted weather situations along the transport route?
- Is the weight of the patient (plus the weight of required equipment and transport personnel) within allowable ranges for air transport?
- For inter-hospital transports, is there a helipad and/or airport near the referring hospital?
- Does the patient require critical care life support (e.g., monitoring personnel, specific medications, and specific equipment) during transport, which is not available with ground transport options?
- Would use of local ground transport leave the local area without adequate emergency medical services coverage?
- If local ground transport is not an option, can the needs of the patient (and the system) be met by an available regional ground critical care transport service (i.e., specialized surface transport systems operated by hospitals and/or air medical programs)?

Auto-Launch Programs

Patients with certain life threatening conditions benefit from immediate assistance and rapid intervention. Patients with time critical conditions such as acute multi-system trauma, aortic dissection, myocardial infarction, stroke, and complications associated with labor and delivery benefit from transfers to specialized centers. Many AMS programs develop partnerships with referring partners to shorten the response time in cases where patients meet criteria of the auto-launch program. Once activated, these programs provide automatic response procedures.

These auto launch programs activate a series of procedures designed to minimize the time it takes to dispatch an air medical team to the patient. Most auto-launch programs include procedures that allow the communications center to prioritize the request for service above any other routine transfer and make immediate arrangements such as:

- Connect the referring clinicians or agencies directly to the accepting service.
- Make a bed available in the proper hospital area for the patient
- Communicate with the pilot in command for approval of the flight request
- Dispatch the air medical team
- Coordinate with the referring agency or facility to arrange for landing zone support
- Arrange any ground transportation necessary to move the medical team and the patient if the aircraft cannot land at the scene or facility.

A recent paper out of Japan[10] characterized the time savings appreciated when AMS dispatch was included in the response to a crash detected by automatic crash detection sensors installed in modern automobiles.

8.7 POLICY AND PROCEDURAL ISSUES

Ground Transport to the Referring Facility or Accident/Disaster Scene

Ground transport of the medical team and the patient may be required on one or both legs of a transport in situations where the aircraft cannot reach the patient's location to within walking distance. This may be due to a lack of a suitable helipad on site or hazards in the area which prevent safe operation of the aircraft.

Incident Command

Air medical programs frequently respond to requests for service from other public safety agencies. Each program must account the way its team members interact and coordinate with the requesting agency. Most public safety agencies appoint a scene or incident commander for each accident or disaster scene. This person bears responsibility for coordination and oversight of the entire response. Air medical teams represent a precious medical resource and therefore should communicate with the incident commander or their delegate as to thes best use of their skills and capacity.

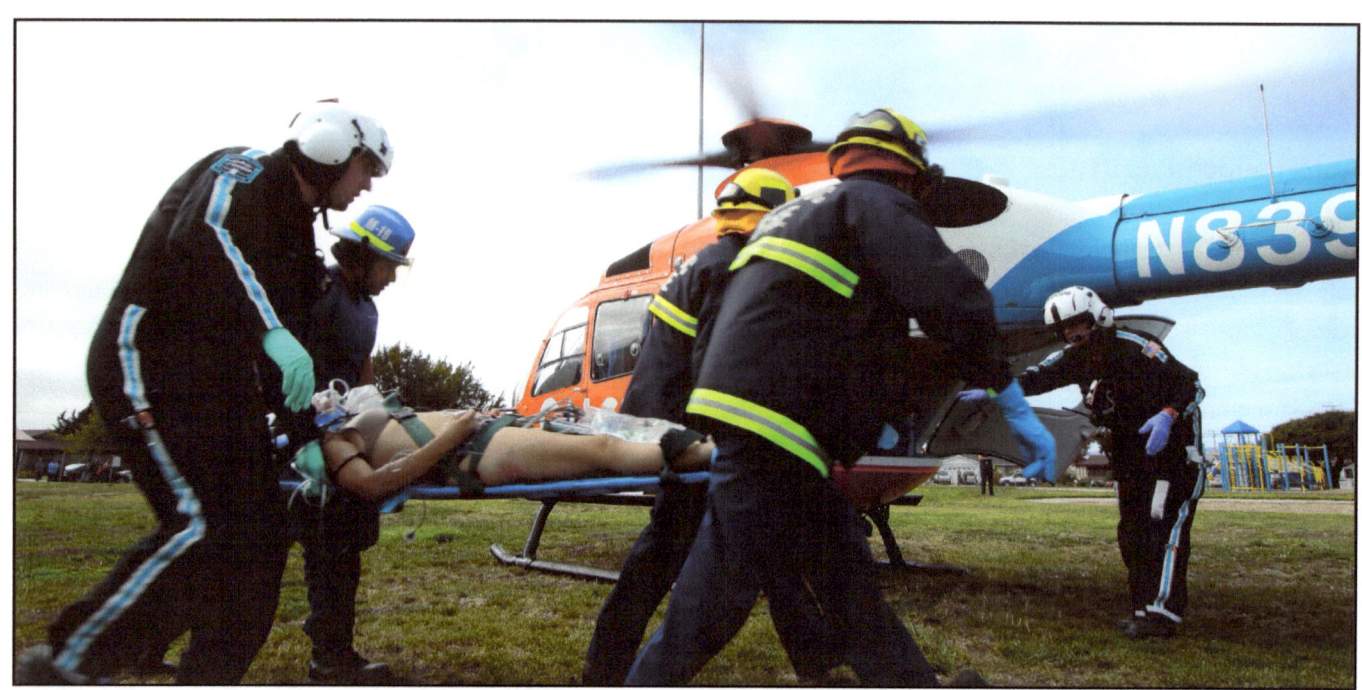

Photo courtesy of Mark Mennie Photography

Pilot Assistance

While the pilot bears primary responsibility for the safe operation and security of the aircraft, some pilots will also aid the medical crew in carrying equipment or moving the patient. Many pilots prefer direct involvement in patient loading to assure the safe and secure positioning of the patient within the aircraft.

Additional Patients & Family

Decisions to transport additional patients or family members of the primary patient depend on the nature of the injuries, the intensity of care required, the carrying capacity of the airframe and pilot recommendations for safety. The pilot in command has the final decision on this matter.

Law Enforcement Attendant

In some cases, a patient may be attended to by law enforcement officials prior to and during the transport. Each program develops its own policies and procedure related to the carrying of firearms in the aircraft and the management of patient restraints and handcuffs in the case of potentially dangerous or violent patients.

Patient Treatment Prior to Take Off

The confined space and movement of the aircraft make certain delicate medical procedures more difficult. Many air medical professionals modify procedures and develop unique strategies to facilitate the performance of invasive procedures. In most cases, truly invasive procedures are performed prior to entering the aircraft.

These may include:

- Intubation or surgical cricothyroidotomy
- Chest tubes
- Insertion of central and/or arterial lines
- Interosseous lines

Securing Equipment & the Patient

The aircraft and its occupants experience a great deal of movement during the trip. Secure storage of all medical equipment and snug but comfortable seatbelt application to the patient prevent accidents and injury in the event of sudden changes in direction or altitude.

Communication with the Patient

Noise and vibration make verbal and physical communication with the patient difficult. Awake patients may be offered headsets connected to the crew's communication link to keep the patient informed of the status of the trip and inquire about any ongoing pain or concerns of the patient.

Patient Treatments En Route

While most emergency procedures are best performed prior to transport, sometimes a patient's condition changes during the trip. Medical crews and pilots must be prepared to respond quickly to stabilize any emergency conditions. In some cases, an emergency situation may occur that requires a change in altitude or the destination of the flight. Pilots and medical crews must be able to discuss the situation and determine the best response to the situation. Each member of the team must provide appropriate medical care during the flight.

En Route Care Includes the following:

- Resuscitation
- Airway management – Intubation, Oxygen therapy, airway suctioning, cricothyroidotomy
- Invasive procedures
- Adjustment of therapy
- Monitoring of patient vital signs
- Point of care lab testing for chemistry, blood counts and blood gases
- Blood products
- Medication Administration
- Vasoactive agents
- Cardiopulmonary Resuscitation including chest compressions
- Management of life support equipment, (monitors, IV pumps, suction, oxygen supply, LVAD, ECMO, intra-aortic balloon pumps, ventilators, etc.)

Communication with the Receiving Institution Regarding the Patient's Needs

Clinical communication between all stakeholders should be early, open, and comprehensive. This starts from the earliest 'referral call'; from the calling hospital (inter-hospital) or emergency response services (pre-hospital). While inter-hospital and pre-hospital clinical communication is inherently very different, the principles are the same. Relevant, early communication to the likely 'down-stream' services should occur. For inter-hospital referrals, engaging a clinical discussion with the referring clinicians to optimize and enhance local care can be highly beneficial. In some cases, engagement with referral clinicians (destination hospital and/or specific specialist services such as burns, toxicology, neonatal, or pediatric intensive care) can identify patients who with appropriate advice may be safely triaged to simpler transfer strategies; including no transfer.

Obviously if there are financial pressures to move patients, this is harder to achieve. In systems that are not dependent on such activity for their viability, such triaging mechanisms reduce the opportunity cost of having a HEMS response unavailable for the patients for whom HEMS has the greatest efficacy. The communications should, ideally, be direct and multi-party. Referring and referral clinicians should be able to discuss the patient with the medical direction of the potential transport solution represented in that conference call.

8.8 OPERATING IN MILITARY-CONTROLLED OR CONFLICT ZONES

Conflict/Military Zones

Conflict zones require coordination with military movement command and control center to avoid both "friendly" and enemy fire, as well as direct coordination with the people on the ground, which can be chaotic, to ensure landing at the correct location at the correct time, often involving a grid locations and colored smoke indicator. Another factor is coordinating with local civilian air space authorities which concede control of air-space to the military. For remote medical evacuations, a security team may need to be ready for suppression-fire and securing the perimeter upon landing.

Security Planning and Operations

Operating in a conflict zone or active war zone requires coordination with, and sanctioned support from, the organization or governing military organization controlling the airspace. Typically, operations will be employed by this same governing military organization. In addition, coordination with civilian air traffic controller both directly and through the military is necessary. Additional risks will be present since there is conflict with insurgents; for this reason, intelligence reports are necessary for any flight planning which often be only "need to know" information. Conflict zones can be chaotic and military personnel in the field expect an adaptable, results driven approach with less bureaucratic "red-tape".

Situations can become even more confusing with multiple groups like the United Nations / UNHAS, NATO, Russian Federation (Ukraine and Syria), African Union, etc. in addition to the home country's Ministry of Defense and Ministry of Transport (e.g., Civil Aviation Authority), Airport specific Air Traffic Control. The main point is that personality of the local military command and degree of control over the air-space factors into flight operations in conflict zones and this all must be managed to fly safely, especially in an emergency EMS situation.

The first step is to get to know the military command managing flights and air space and understand how they want you to operate. There should be a Government Flight Representative (GFR) assigned to your operation to ensure proper support, coordination and safe operations. There will be standard operating procedures and reference materials for known landing zones in addition to unique procedures and specialized training for the military and specific to the location for crew and non-crew personnel. Below are some standard requirements in a military controlled operation.

Flight Planning

- Flight planning area, weather forecast and intelligence reports
- Flight profiles detailing planned flight checks and events, proficiency training, geographical details and point to point routes, procedures to maximize ground radar monitoring, radio communications, status report intervals, chase aircraft status.
- Flight approval with clear procedures by GFR to ensure seamless support and coordination with Government flights and operations.
- Flight Supervision to ensure crew and aircraft qualification, communications with both military command and local authorities (CAA / FAA air traffic control, safety and maintenance checks, evaluations

Airfield Operations

- Flight profiles detailing planned flight checks and events, proficiency training, geographical details
- Compliance with directives and execute any agreements with airfield authority to ensure full compliance
- Qualifications and certification requirements for radio operators or tower controllers
- Weather Requirements for ceiling/visibility minimums and alternate weather requirements
- Understanding flight operating limits
- Filing of flight plans
- Arming policies and requirements
- Daylight or night vision / low light operations requirements
- Emergency operating procedures with attention to radio failure, landing gear malfunctions, in-flight fire, emergency fuel procedures to name of a few.
- Aircrew briefing / debriefing, weight and balance determination, fuel requirements

Ground Operations

- Develop procedures including housekeeping, flight line vehicle operation, selection, training, testing, certifying of personnel in all normal and emergency operations
- Foreign object damage prevention program and procedures
- Procedures for hazardous materials, munitions, fueling and related operations, towing, lifting devices, oxygen, work stands, maintenance/inspection methods and standards, auxiliary power units, gearbox and other servicing procedures, tool control, storage of oil, lubricants, oxygen, etc.
- Severe weather plans
- Training requirements for ground personnel and evaluation procedures

Operational Consideration

- Protocols for Military and Dual-Use Airports
- Communications: UHF vs VHF, Satcom
- Military Logging and Documentation requirements

Below is an example of a Concept of Operations (Conop) typical for a US Army operation in Afghanistan:

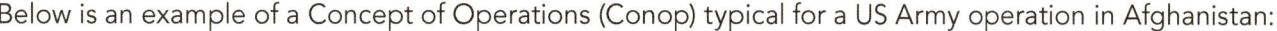

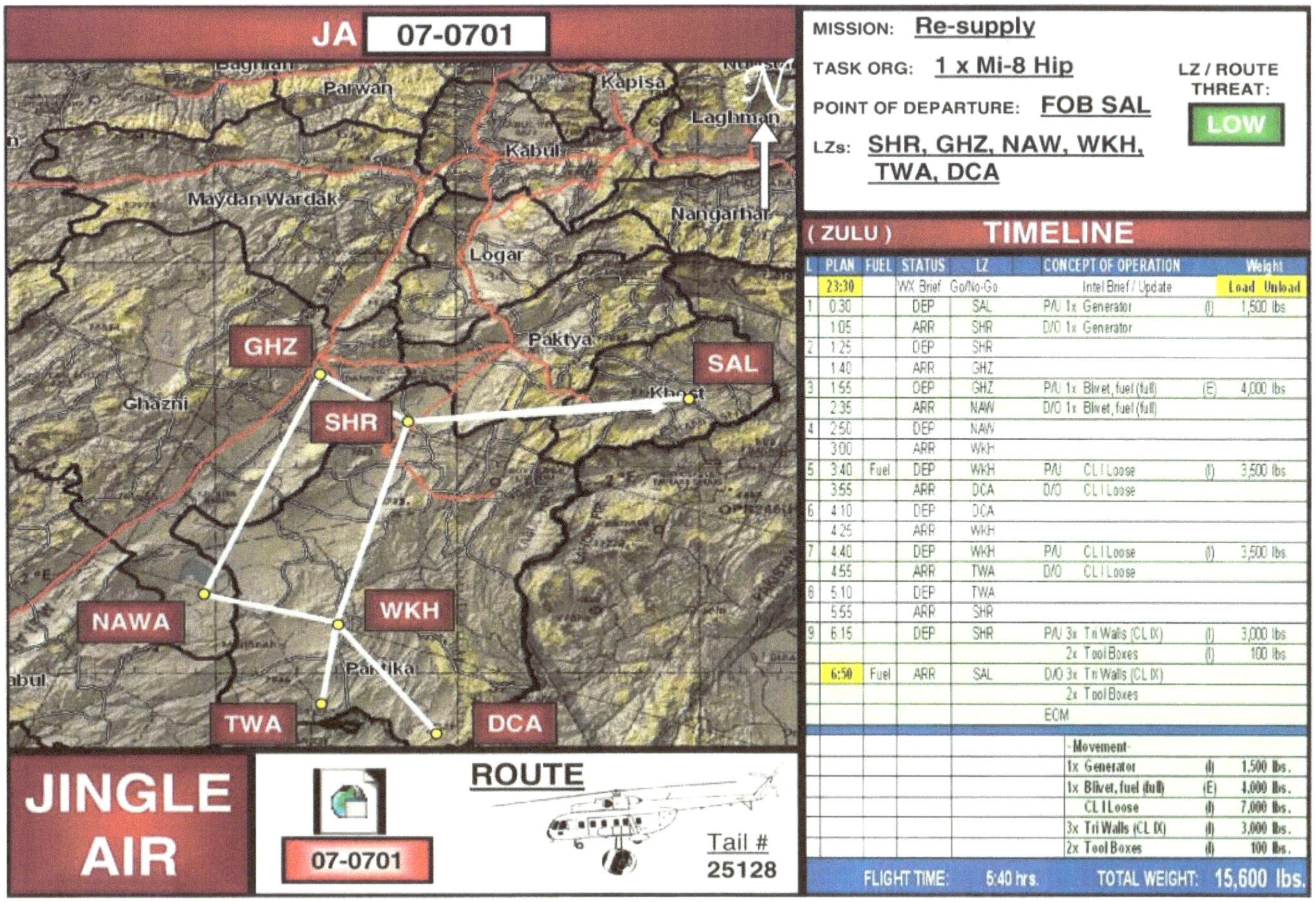

Medical Considerations

- Personnel
- Pharmaceuticals
- Medical Logging and Documentation requirements

Aviation Safety Program

- Mishap prevention program for both flight and ground operations
- Establish Flight Safety person responsible training, procedures, safety audits, assessments, reports, currency, and documentation of all regular meetings
- Mishap Response Plan detailing policies, responsibilities, actions

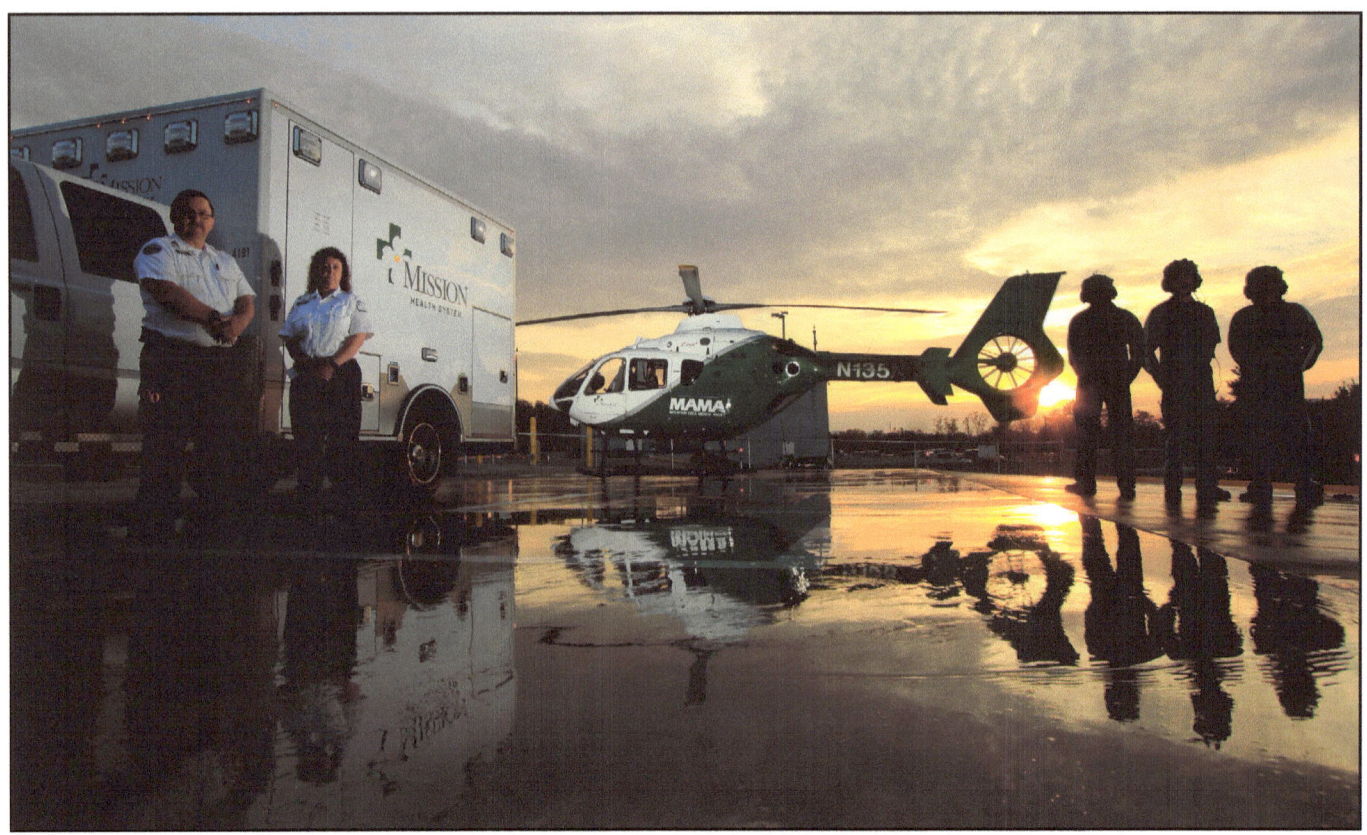

Photo courtesy of Mark Mennie Photography

Expect the Unexpected

Coordinating a civilian operation into a military theater under military command will generate unexpected challenges and there will be ambiguous grey areas that may require subtle management to avoid problems. In general, include your GFR with your problems and issues to help resolve issues.

Here are a few examples:

- Dealing with corrupt airport officials asking for bribes for parking aircraft and facing problems when the corrupt officials do not get what they want. This may happen in a joint civilian / military airport when the military does not have space in their territory. The military often will not engage corruption from the host nation and may offer no help. And if you are foolish enough to break the law and support corruption and are caught, do not naively expect the military to support you.
- Receiving compromised fuel in a remote refueling location managed by the military. The lesson is that remote locations sometimes lack quality and procedures which are expected in the main military bases.
- Aircraft taking fire, compromising performance in an area that is too hostile / dangerous to remain
- Arming needs that are supported by the military but possibly not supported by the host nation
- Dealing with a bureaucratic military slow to fix and/or address problems like dust suppression

- Fly-overs by military aircraft like Chinook helicopters (CH-47) doing damage to your helicopters. Even if unnecessary, do not expect all military pilots to behave and do not expect the military to compensate for damage to your aircraft
- The interface, especially in a new conflict zone or one with multiple stakeholders, may be confusing and unclear. Initiative and forcing the stakeholders to take a stand that provide clarity is important. The rules and methods are often developing and more fluid than in a mature conflict zone

CHAPTER 9

Air Medical Program Administration

9.1 INTRODUCTION

Air medical programs require the coordinated effort of a wide range of professional and support staff. Most programs appoint a leadership team. The leadership team provides the direction, oversight, and procedural guidance that enables the members of the service to perform their duties. This team usually includes experienced medical, aviation, and administrative personnel. The leadership team overseas the day to day operation of the service and creates the conditions in which the service members perform their roles.

The leadership team creates the organization's structure and function. They assign roles, responsibilities, positions, titles, and reporting structures to accomplish all of the necessary aspects of the service. The leadership team determines the policies and procedures consistent with the mission of the service.

This leadership holds all members of the service accountable for adhering to the legal and regulatory guidance of outside agencies. They provide support and corrective actions for their staff to maintain the mission. Continuously interact with stakeholders and patients to ensure the programs remains relevant and responsive to the needs of the patients, communities, and partners they serve.

Many programs create an administrative team to handle the many non-medical and non-aviation functions associated with air medical services. These administrative teams can have more or fewer layers depending on whether the program stands alone or functions within a larger institution or agency.

9.2 BUSINESS OPERATIONS

Like any organization or business, air medical services perform the same routine business functions associated with operating a service. While the complexity of these functions may vary depending on the business model in use, all AMS programs perform the routine business operations including:

Air medical services, whether for-profit or otherwise, must engage in business relationships and activities with customers, payers, suppliers, and specialized vendors and the public. These relationships require ongoing attention to contracting, invoicing, budgeting, bill paying, supply chain management, logistics, real estate, marketing, information services, controlled access storage, accounting and reporting of accounts. Every program must manage its business activities according to its business model and the locally prevailing laws and codes that apply. Staff must be experienced in the multitude of processes and laws governing the conduct of business in the areas where the air medical service operates.

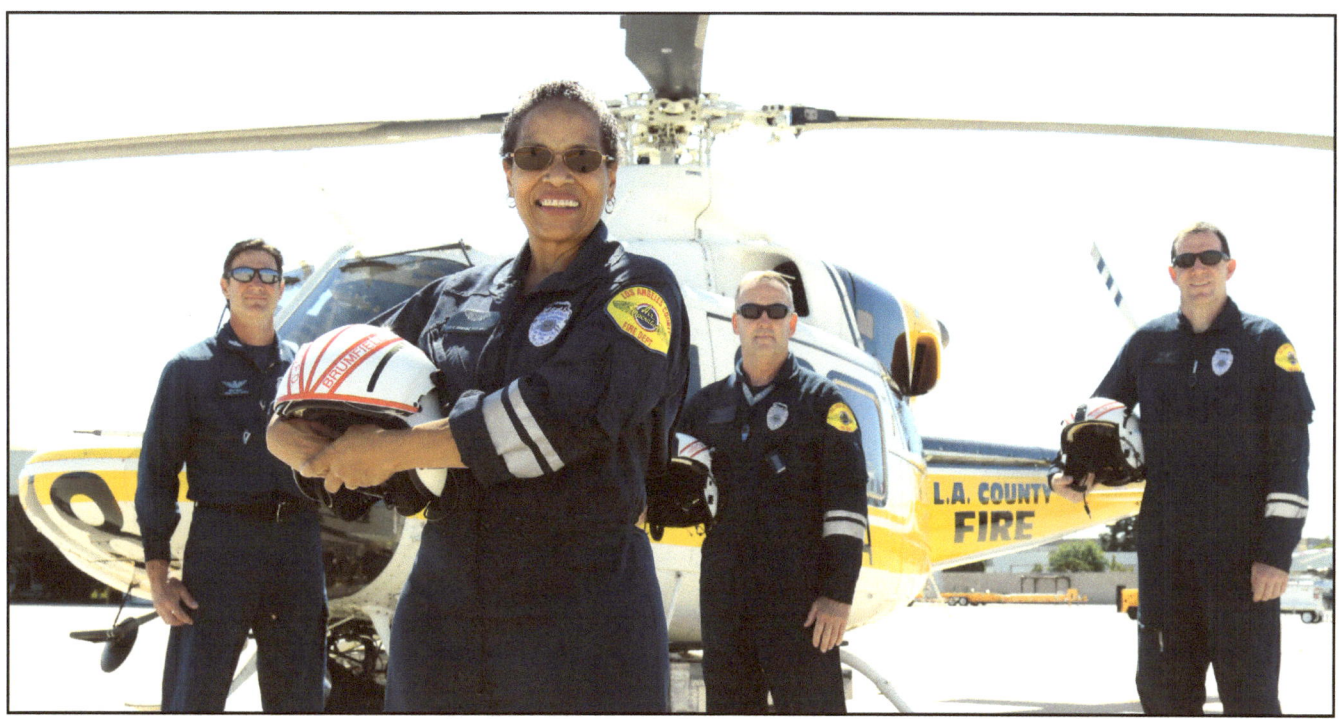

Photo courtesy of Mark Mennie Photography

9.3 STAFFING, TRAINING & HUMAN RESOURCES

Managing the recruitment, retention & replacement and payment of the air medical service's staff along with maintaining the schedules, training requirements, certification processes requires a full range of human resource management knowledge and expertise. All programs expend significant time and energy in recruiting, retaining and replacing the necessary experts and support staff to operate the service. All staff members, regardless of their role, require training and familiarization time to integrate into the culture and work flow of the service.

Since air medical services typically operate 24 hours per day, staffing requirements typically match those of other round the clock services. Most rotor wing programs medical crews work 12 to 24 hour shifts, while fixed wing programs may need to consider staffing models that account for multi-day missions in the case of international repatriation flights. These staffing requirements extend to dispatch, administrative and support personnel as well. Staffing the service for 24 hours a day operations requires that programs account for the scheduling of mission specific pilot and medical crew training along with any legally mandated corporate and safety training for the entire crew. In many cases, dispatchers, communications specialists, coders, billers, and maintenance personnel also require ongoing training and recertification relevant to their respective roles.

Every air medical program requires teams of pilots, dispatchers, communications specialists, medical staff, mechanics, avionics support, administrative, legal & clerical support, billing specialists and public relations staff. Many programs use the services of both part-time and full-time employees and independent contractors and vendors daily. Like any employed person they require all the support typically associated with working a job including schedules, oversight, accountability, clearly defined responsibilities, reporting structures, & compensation.

9.4 MARKETING AND PUBLIC RELATIONS

Air medical programs enjoy a relatively high profile amongst emergency response services. Helicopters and medical rescue teams generate significant excitement wherever they go. The high profile comes with a responsibility to maintain a professional and positive appearance. Everything an air medical program and its personnel does impacts its reputation and sends a message to the patients, payers, partners and general public about the spirit and capability of the program.

Each member of the air medical service represents the service itself. The attitudes and professionalism of the staff along with the appearance of the aircraft, uniforms, and marketing materials all affect the perception of the service amongst the various people and institutions they serve. Marketing occurs with every patient encounter, conversation with family, interaction with other first responders and clinicians, along with the more formal messaging released via internet, video, print media outlets and news services.

Public Relations Events

Many programs deliver specific public relations events as part of their ongoing marketing efforts. These range from having the helicopter land at public events, to staff providing education and training to public safety personnel and the general public on health or safety related topics. Some programs sponsor formal continuing medical education events to encourage better relationships with referring and receiving clinicians and institutions. Still others sponsor a variety of fundraising events to create opportunities for the public to engage the service directly and fund specific program needs.

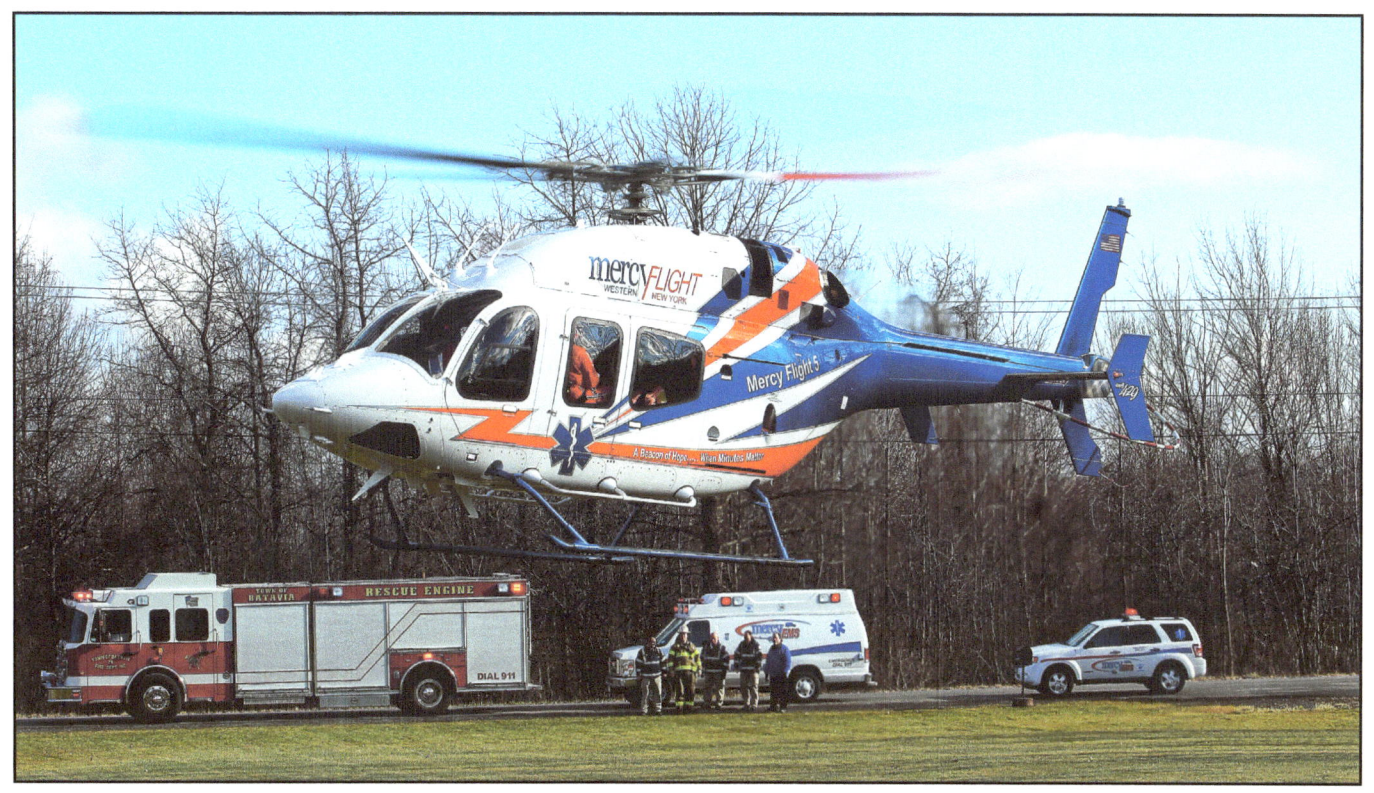

Photo provided by Bell Helicopter, A Textron Company

9.5 INTEGRATION INTO THE LOCAL HEALTHCARE SYSTEM

Integrating the air medical program into an existing healthcare system requires advanced planning, careful training, and ongoing communication with the referring and receiving facilities. Integration occurs as a continuous process with three phases.

The initial phase occurs during the planning process as shown in the logic model. Simply asking people and healthcare workers about their attitudes and willingness to use an air medical system plants the idea in their minds. Coming back to them with additional questions and information will allow the program to begin shaping its relationship to these people and the institutions they support.

The second phase begins when the program begins to develop and train the air medical teams. It can be useful to engage the local media at this point, offering interviews and allowing reporters to observe and report on the program and its training efforts. Additional outreach through public relations events, landing zone training, drills, and simulated missions involving referring agencies and hospital staff allows prospective users and current stakeholders to interact with the program and become familiar with its operations.

The third phase includes all of the ongoing interactions, communication, marketing, and quality assurance activities that make up the totality of the program. This phase begins with the first patient transport and continues indefinitely for the life of the program. A successful program continuously monitors and maintains the relationships with potential and current users and adjust its activities to maintain its relevance to the needs of the patients and providers who serve them.

9.6 MEDICAL EQUIPMENT AND MEDICAL SUPPLIES

Air medical programs provide a broad range of medical and surgical care to patients in remote locations. Since air medical teams move to the patient, they must bring their equipment with them. Most air medical programs rely on a carry enough medication and equipment to care for a critically ill patient, and one or more non-critical patients. Most teams select and organize their equipment based on how often they use various tools and weight and durability. Most programs develop kits based on the typical medical scenarios they encounter and the capabilities of the medical crew. Further, most programs use patient monitors, ventilators, and supplies developed for use in out of hospital environments and EMS.

Air medical operations use a wide spectrum of technically sophisticated equipment both in the aircraft themselves and the medical suite onboard. All programs must be prepared for the ongoing process of acquiring the necessary equipment and supplies used by the service. From airplanes to bandages, each item used in air medical services has a life cycle that includes acquisition times, and the necessity of proper storage and use, routine maintenance, repair, useful life cycles, updates and replacement.

All medical equipment requires inspection, certification, recalibration and ongoing control testing on a regular basis. Maintaining and replacing damaged or defective equipment on schedule or in time for the next transport requires close coordination between budgeting, maintenance activities and acquisition processes to allow the air medical program to function smoothly

Each piece of equipment has its own life cycle, with varying time frames associated with acquisition, maintenance schedules, maintenance, calibration and replacement. Most programs track and log these activities to demonstrate and track performance as well as predict when equipment must be taken out of service or replaced. Since much of the equipment requires specialized expertise to maintain, most programs establish relationships with experts in the aviation industry, medical supply houses, specific equipment vendors and biomedical engineering to assist them in maintaining the variety of equipment used during their work.

9.7 PHARMACEUTICALS

Modern healthcare relies heavily on pharmaceutical therapies. Air medical providers typically carry a wide array of emergency cardiac and vasoactive medications as well as enough IV fluids to resuscitate a critically ill trauma patient. The extent to which the program develops its pharmacy program depends on local regulatory requirements, supply chain issues, and the needs of the patients they serve.

9.8 LABORATORY

The past decade has seen tremendous developments in bedside laboratory testing technology. It is now possible to perform rapid assessments of metabolic, respiratory and cardiac markers in the field. Many air medical teams now deploy with handheld analyzers capable of providing reliable analysis of blood with cartridge based blood testing for blood counts, chemistries, blood gases, blood types and certain infectious diseases. Local conditions, temperature, and altitude all affect the reliability of these products and cost represents a significant determinant for inclusion in a program's load out.

9.9 BLOOD PRODUCTS AND BLOOD BANKING

Some air medical programs provide un-cross matched blood products as part of their therapeutic armamentarium. Access to blood banks, temperature controlled transport cases and the proper administration sets allow a team to initiate blood transfusions while en route. Blood banking facilities and strict adherence to quality and safety procedures ensure the blood remains available, viable and safe for patients who need it.

9.10 MEDICAL RECORDS

The medical crew creates the medical record in accordance with local regulations and reimbursement requirements. Paper printouts and handwritten forms often suffice. Today, with the advent of portable electronic devices and medical charting software, many programs create electronic medical records of each patient encounter. Some software programs integrate the medical chart directly into the entire transport record alongside the flight and administrative records.

Regardless of the method of record keeping, each patient encounter requires adequate documentation. Each record serves as a communication tool to convey medical information and a record of the transport for such diverse purposes as coding, billing, collections, database construction, medical oversight and quality assurance.

9.11 CLEANUP, WASTE HANDLING, BIOHAZARD DISPOSAL

Patient care always generates soiled linens, contaminated medical supplies, sharp waste and discarded packaging. Most medical crews participate in cleaning the airframe and crew compartments after each transport. Many programs develop standard cleaning and stocking checklists which crews follow immediately after every trip. The entire team must ensure a clean, well-stocked and fully functioning aircraft prior to the next call for service.

Most governments regulate the disposal of contaminated medical waste. Many programs contract with licensed disposal firms or develop in-house waste and cleaning programs to meet the various regulatory and health and safety standards.

Returning Equipment from other Medical Services

Air medical services routinely interface with other medical institutions, public safety agencies and emergency responders. Often during patient care, a medical provider from one agency or institution may apply a medical device or tool that must stay with the patient for the duration of the transport. In some cases, those devices are reusable and must be returned to the original institution or agency from which it came. Most programs design a process using local package delivery services or postal services to return equipment to the originating service in a timely manner. Attention to promptly returning other service's equipment serves both a positive public relations function and prevents the accumulation of important medical equipment in one location.

CHAPTER 10

Air Medical Program Accreditation

10.1 PROGRAM EVALUATION

Once local, regional or national regulations are met, programs can move beyond regulatory requirements established by government agency responsible for air medical programs to achieve operational validation through 3rd party accreditation.

10.2 THIRD PARTY ACCREDITTION

Some air medical programs chose to move beyond simple compliance with regulatory requirements programs to achieve operational validation through third party accreditation. Accreditation allows a program to tell its customers that the program meets specific standards for service and can be expected and relied upon to meet the minimum necessary standards of the accrediting body. This allows for a higher level of confidence in the quality and safety of a program for clients and potential customers.

Generally, compliance with accreditation standards is measured on an ongoing basis by the accrediting organization. The accreditation standards are periodically revised to reflect the advancement and changing environment of air medical transport with considerable input from all disciplines of the medical profession. Each organization can provide prospective programs with specific criteria and process information.

The benefits of third party accreditation include:

- Increased attention to safety practices
- Improved documentation of processes and systems
- Fewer licensing issues
- Compliance with regulatory guidelines
- Competitive advantage in contracting
- Opportunities for marketing
- Lower liability insurance costs
- Decreases legal liability costs in litigation
- Quality Management Systems

A major part of third-party accreditation involves the use of formalized quality management systems. These systems allow programs to deliver the best possible service and make improvements as a normal part of their work. Each quality management system uses various standards, measures of performance, benchmarks and feedback processes to ensure that each aspect of the air medical program delivers the specific best outcomes and meets the predetermined goals set forward in the standards they adopt.

Some public and private entities may require third party accreditation as a precondition for forming partnerships or assigning contracts for service. In some cases, the specific client performs the accreditation process themselves. For example, programs seeking to partner with the United Nations must undergo a thorough operational audit and inspection prior to engaging the UN for consideration as a partner.

Accreditation standards also serve as a guide in the development of the air medical program as it relates to quality, safety, administration, and overall operations even if a program is not seeking accreditation at the time. The accreditation process often assists programs in identifying areas of strength and areas for improvement. The use of formal quality management systems and the industry standards allows new programs to describe and evaluate the quality of their service.

Below are three commonly used accreditation services, each of which provide certifications domestically and internationally. Some air medical programs may choose to obtain accreditation from more than one organization, depending on the requirements of stakeholders, clients, governments and other partners.

10.3 CAMTS - COMMISSION ON ACCREDITATION OF MEDICAL TRANSPORT SYSTEMS

www.camts.org

The Commission on Accreditation of Medical Transport Systems (CAMTS), is an independent, non-profit service which audits and accredits fixed-wing and rotary wing air medical transport services, as well as ground inter-facility critical care services, to a set of industry-established criteria. CAMTS is an organization of non-profit organizations dedicated to improving the quality and safety of medical transport services, with 21 current member organizations each of which sends one representative to the CAMTS Board of Directors.

Originally developed through an extensive public comment process and published in 1991, revised every 2-3 years, the Accreditation Standards address issues of patient care and safety in fixed and rotary wing services as well as ground inter-facility services providing critical care transports. Each standard is supported by measurable criteria to measure a program's level of quality.

CAMTS offers a program of voluntary evaluation of compliance with accreditation standards demonstrating the ability to deliver service of a specific quality.

10.4 NAAMTA - NATIONAL ACCREDITATION ALLIANCE, MEDICAL TRANSPORT APPLICATIONS

www.naamta.com

NAAMTA provides accreditation services to ground and air medical transport organizations worldwide. With an ISO 9001:2008 Certified Quality Management System, NAAMTA works with its client organizations to build successful programs that are accredited to a high level of internationally-recognized standards.

NAAMTA partners with its members in the form of an alliance to continue to support their program development and operations. NAAMTA provides accreditation and program audits services and assist their members in developing robust quality management and training support. The alliance members also benefit from information sharing, online documentation tools, and online training and education.

NAAMTA promotes a non-punitive, transparent, objective and measurable process that allows for continuous quality improvement. On-going support is provided via web and personal interactions.

10.5 EURAMI - EUROPEAN AIR MEDICAL INSTITUTE

www.eurami.org

Based in Germany, the European Air Medical Institute (EURAMI) provides third party accreditation, advocacy, and support to air medical services throughout Europe and the world. Their services cover both fixed and rotor-wing aircraft.

EURAMI advocates for high quality air rescue and emergency care for all patients and promote the provision of scientifically validated medical care to regardless of their age, gender, race, religion, or philosophy of life.

EURAMI's services include consultancy, lobbying, accreditation, research & development, as well as networking.

CHAPTER 11

Air Medical Education and Training Programs

1. Formal education and training for EMS pilots
2. Formal air medical education and training programs for medical providers
3. Ride along programs
4. LZ educational programs for EMS

11.1 MEDICAL TEAM TRAINING

Recruiting and training medical team members to deliver the highest quality care in the air medical environment requires dedicated educational resources and involves a significant financial commitment. As the demand for highly trained air medical providers continues to increase, universities and private organizations have responded by creating specialized certificate and graduate level training in air medical services. Partnerships between HEMS programs and university based nursing and medicine programs represent a pipeline for manpower development and ongoing training and assessment. On-line continuing education has become more accessible and affordable offering updates on the latest trends in patient care, safety, leadership, aviation and more.

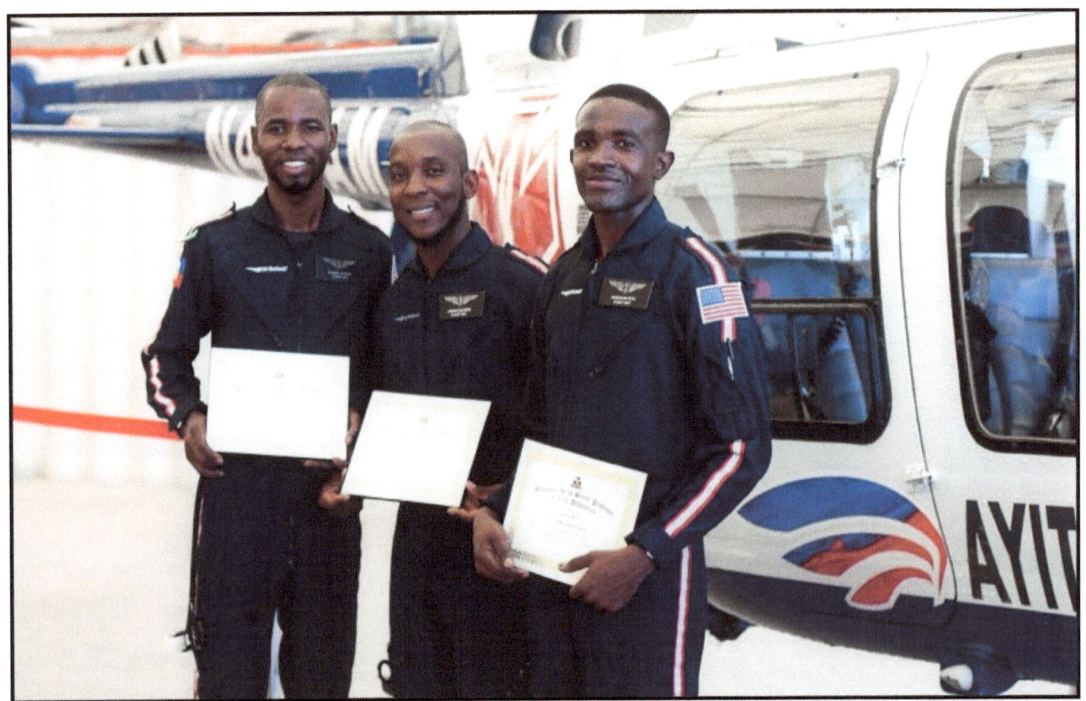

Photo courtesy of Haiti Air Ambulance

Many programs[1,2] have developed realistic simulator training for their medical teams. Examples include the use of high fidelity patient simulators, mock disaster drills, water egress training devices and full motion flight simulators, in addition to traditional laboratory classes, hospital rotations and operating room experience-building.

For example, STARS in Calgary, as well as other programs, converted recreational vehicles into a mobile training service with a human patient simulator that can be programmed to replicate signs and symptoms of complex medical and traumatic conditions such as difficult airway management, traumatic brain injury, cardiac failure with a mannequin that speaks, breathes, blinks, reactive pupils, palpable pulses and more, all in the setting of either an aircraft or in the emergency room.

11.2 JOINT MEDICAL AND FLIGHT CREW TRAINING

Training pilots and medical teams to work together to manage the entire mission requires specialized facilities. In the past programs relied on mentorship and on-the-job training. It could take many years for a crewmember to accumulate the experience necessary to function independently as a team leader. Today, there are dedicated simulation centers in Europe and the U.S. using retired helicopter fuselages and high fidelity patient simulators to train medical and aviation team members in realistic scenarios. It is now possible to expose trainees to a wide range of clinical and operational conditions to build experience and shorten the time it take to gain competency in the core skills and procedures necessary to safely and effectively operate in the air medical environment. Even water emergency egress training can now be done safely and simply using a roll cage and a pool. A great deal of cross-training occurs naturally as each member of the team gains experience. Training together enhances interpersonal relationships, builds confidence, and allows for enhanced team situation awareness.

11.3 TRAINING FACILITIES AND PROGRAMS

Full service air medical training facilities now exist in many parts of the world. Each program serves a broad geographic region and focuses on providing as much realistic hands on training in air medical services. These facilities typically include state of the art simulation, allowing students exposure to many different scenarios to increase their experience in air medical services. Below are a few examples of full service air medical training facilities.

The Dorothy Ebersbach Academic Center for Flight Nursing at Case Western Reserve University – U.S.
https://case.edu/nursing/flight/

In the U.S. the Dorothy Ebersbach Academic Center for Flight Nursing at Case Western Reserve University in Cleveland Ohio began operating an air medical flight simulator in 2015.[3] They converted a retired Sikorsky S-76 fuselage into a full motion simulator with enhanced video graphics and high-fidelity flight simulation. It is housed in a state of the art educational facility that includes complete video, sound, and data recording capability as well as classrooms and multi-purpose space. They can simulate a variety of flight conditions and put medical teams through intense clinical scenarios using high-fidelity human patient simulators.

ADAC HEMS Academy - Germany
http://www.hems-academy.de/en/

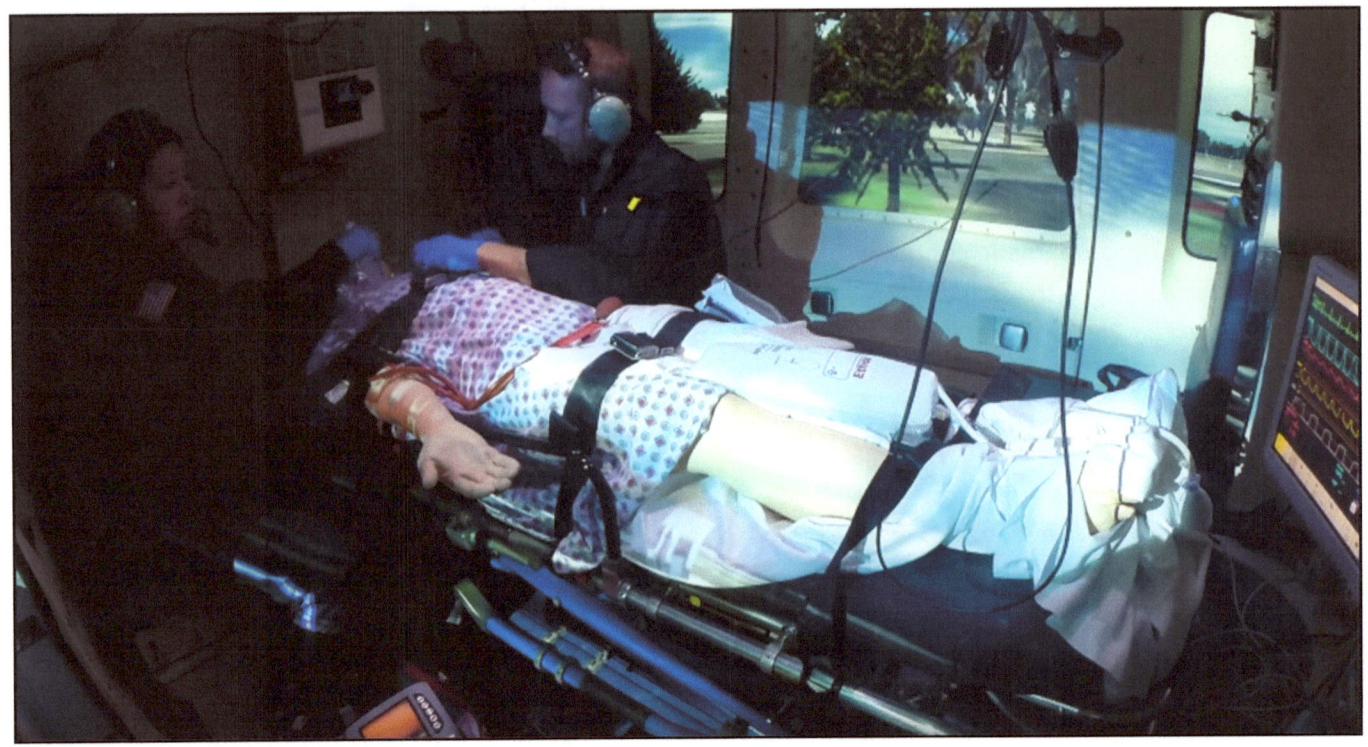

Photo courtesy of Dorothy Ebersbach Academic Center for Flight Nursing, Case Western Reserve University

The German ADAC HEMS Academy began training air medical operators in Sankt Augustin near Cologne-Bonn Airport in July 2009. It is considered the world's first fully integrated training center for HEMS pilots, emergency doctors, and rescue paramedics. The facility provides training and briefing rooms, two full-motion Christoph Sim simulators (EC 135 and EC 145), and state-of-the-art technology including human patient computerized simulators. The ADAC HEMS Academy uses a retired EC 135 fuselage for training. They offer scenarios such as patient transfer between helicopter crew and accepting hospital team, challenging patient care cases, and much more. Trainers follow students via one-way mirrors and record each training session for teaching and debriefing purposes.

The HEMS Academy also offers pilots mandatory flight simulation training and mission specific coursework in topics including confined space, off-shore, and mountainous terrain operations. Training with the medical team optimizes air medical crew resource management and team situation awareness.

RACQ CareFlight – Australia
http://www.lifeflight.org.au/page/what-we-do/lifeflight-training-services/

RACQ CareFlight recently announced a partnership with Aviation Australia which will reimburse CareFlight for $15,000 per year worth of underwater escape training at Aviation Australia's Brisbane Airport. With an additional $15,000 donated by 50 Aviation Australia employees, CareFlight is equipping its aviation and medical teams with the practical knowledge that could save their lives should an aircraft have an emergency landing in the water. Numerous programs across the world have adopted this technique to train their own crews in water egress procedures.

AAMS – Medical Transport Leadership Institute (MTLI) - U.S. and locations worldwide
http://aams.org/events/mtli/

The Institute provides continuing education and certification for individuals currently managing medical transportation services, those seeking management positions, and others with direct and indirect involvement who desire greater understanding of the air medical profession.

Students gain expertise and practical skills through formal didactic and participatory sessions designed to instill creative thinking and decision-making. Participants also obtain valuable insight into real life challenges by networking with industry leaders. The Institute operates with a rigorous approach to competency-based education, utilizing formal classroom hours, mandatory student participation, written testing, oral presentations and a code of professional conduct. Graduates of the two year program will receive certification as a Certified Medical Transport Executive.

The AAMS – Medical Transport Leadership Institute has attracted attendees from over 49 states and the District of Columbia, and 8 international locations. Registrants have included:

- Program Directors/CEOs
- Medical Crew Supervisors
- Emergency Department Supervisors
- Directors of Operations
- Site/Area Managers
- Operators
- Communications Supervisors
- EMS Coordinators
- Hospital Administrators
- Medical Directors
- Directors of Maintenance
- Lead Pilots
- CFOs & Billing Specialists
- Safety Officers

11.4 FULL MISSION PROFILE AND SIMULATIONS

Training with simulations represent a cost-effective and efficient way to introduce new skills to providers. It can also allow a new service to begin interacting with the healthcare system. Table top exercises and dry-runs using simulated patients allow the air medical teams to practice their jobs. In addition, by integrating the exercises into the functioning healthcare system with mock transports and allow healthcare workers to practice interacting with the service and begin integrating it into their referral and response practices. It also allows the service to identify any challenges or obstacles to manage prior to starting patient care activities.

11.5 HEALTH CARE SYSTEM TRAINING

Training healthcare workers and administrators in the use of the air medical service and working with the air medical teams can show significant improvements in utilization and integration of the air medical service into routine healthcare operations.

If hoist/winch operations are part of the mission profile, ongoing training is vital for the safety of the aviation and medical team, as well as the patient and the providers offering scene support. In Germany the ADAC training center uses a converted BK-117 helicopter fuselage to train teams in air medical services. They suspended the fuselage from crane using steel cables. The fuselage "flies" in a large hanger facility simulating controlled flight. The center offers real-life scenarios in as close to challenging terrain as possible without putting the team or the airframe in danger.   German mountain air rescue, military, ADAC and DRF Air Rescue all take part on regular training programs.   Visit: www.bw-zsa.org/simulation for additional information.

Toll and New South Wales Ambulance[4] are building a new combined aviation and medical crew training base in Sydney which includes aviation and medical simulation training, winch training, and helicopter emergency underwater training. Visit: www.bw-zsa.org/simulation for additional information.

11.6 PROFESSIONAL ASSOCIATIONS

Professional continuing education and industry networking opportunities abound at annual and semi-annual industry conferences such as the Air Medical Transport Conference held annually in the U.S., the AirMed Congress held every three years in Europe, and the Aeromedical Society of Australasia (ASA) scientific conference held annually. Additional regional and specialty care conferences that include an air medical component held around the world represent additional venues for accessing high quality clinical practice training and networking.

The Association for Air Medical Services (AAMS) also provides advanced leadership training in a variety of topics with its Medical Transport Leadership Institute.

APPENDIX A

Civilian Aviation Administrations by Region & Country

ALL COUNTRIES

United Nations (UN)   International Civil Aviation Organization
www.icao.int

AFRICA

African Union (AU)   African Civil Aviation Commission
www.afcac.org

Algeria   Directorate of Civil Aviation and Meteorology
www.ministere-transports.gov.dz

Angola   National Civil Aviation Institute
www.inavic.gv.ao

Benin   National Civil Aviation Agency
www.anac.bj

Botswana   Department of Civil Aviation of Botswana
www.dca.gov.bw

Burkina Faso   Agence Nationale de l'Aviation Civile du Burkina Faso
www.anacburkina.org

Burundi   Civil Aviation Authority of Burundi
Tel: +257 2-23707

Cameroon   Cameroon Civil Aviation Authority
www.ccaa.aero

Cape Verde   Agência de Aviação Civil de Cabo Verde
www.aac.cv

Central African Republic	Ministry of Transport and Civil Aviation Tel: +236 615-316
Chad	Autorite de l'Aviation Civile du Tchad www.adac-tchad.org
Comoros	National Agency of Civil Aviation and Meteorology www.anacm-comores.com
Djibouti	Civil Aviation Authority & Meteorology of Djibouti Tel: +253 340-169
DRC - Congo	Autorité de l'Aviation Civile www.aacrdc.org
Republic of the Congo	Agence Nationale de l'Aviation Civile (ANAC Congo) www.anaccongo.org
Egypt	Ministry of Civil Aviation of Egypt www.civilaviation.gov.eg
Equatorial Guinea	Directorate General of Civil Aviation Tel: +240 9-3999
Eritrea	Eritrean Civil Aviation Authority Tel: +291 1-189121
Ethiopia	Ethiopian Civil Aviation Authority www.ecaa.gov.et
Gabon	National Civil Aviation Agency www.anacgabon.org
Gambia	Gambia Civil Aviation Authority www.gambia.gm/gcaa/
Ghana	Ghana Civil Aviation Authority www.gcaa.com.gh
Guinea	Direction Nationale de l'Aviation Civile Guinée Tel: +224 411-928

Guinea-Bissau	Directorate General of Civil Aviation Tel: +245 204-053
Ivory Coast	L'autorité Nationale de l'Aviation Civile (ANAC) www.anac.ci
Kenya	Kenya Civil Aviation Authority www.kcaa.or.ke
Lesotho	Department of Civil Aviation of Lesotho www.civilair.gov.ls
Liberia	Liberia Civil Aviation Authority www.liberiacaa.com
Libya	Libyan Civil Aviation Authority www.caa.gov.ly
Madagascar	Aviation Civile de Madagascar www.acm.mg
Malawi	Department of Civil Aviation of Malawi www.malawi.gov.mw
Mali	Agence Nationale de L'Aviation Civile www.anac-mali.org
Mauritania	l'Agence Nationale de l'Aviation Civile (ANAC) www.anac.mr
Mauritius	Department of Civil Aviation of Mauritius www.civil-aviation.govmu.org
Morocco	Direction Générale de l'Aviation Civile www.dac-maroc.gov.ma/contacter_nous.htm
Mozambique	Civil Aviation Institute of Mozambique www.iacm.gov.mz
Namibia	Directorate of Civil Aviation www.dca.com.na

Niger	l'Agence Nationale de l'Aviation Civile www.anacniger.org
Nigeria	Nigerian Civil Aviation Authority www.ncaa.gov.ng
Rwanda	Rwanda Civil Aviation Authority www.caa.gov.rw
São Tomé and Príncipe	Instituto Nacional de Aviação Civil (INAC) www.inac.st
Senegal	National Civil Aviation Agency of Senegal www.anacim.sn
Seychelles	Seychelles Civil Aviation Authority www.scaa.sc
Sierra Leone	Sierra Leone Civil Aviation Authority (SLCAA) www.slcaa.net
Somalia	Somali Civil Aviation and Meteorology Authority www.scama.so
South Africa	South African Civil Aviation Authority www.caa.co.za
South Sudan	South Sudan Civil Aviation Authority (SSCAA) www.goss.org/index.php/ministries/transport
Sudan	Civil Aviation Authority of Sudan www.caa-sudan.net
Swaziland	Swaziland Civil Aviation Authority (SWACAA) www.swacaa.co.sz
Tanzania	Tanzania Civil Aviation Authority www.tcaa.go.tz
Togo	Civil Aviation Agency of Togo www.anac-togo.tg

Tunisia	Office of Civil Aviation and Airports www.oaca.nat.tn
Uganda	Civil Aviation Authority of Uganda www.caa.co.ug
Zambia	Department of Civil Aviation www.dca.com.zm
Zimbabwe	Civil Aviation Authority of Zimbabwe www.caaz.co.zw

ASIA

China	Civil Aviation Administration of China www.caac.gov.cn
Hong Kong	Civil Aviation Department www.cad.gov.hk
Japan	Japan Civil Aviation Bureau www.mlit.go.jp
Mongolia	Civil Aviation Authority of Mongolia www.mcaa.gov.mn
North Korea (DPRK)	Civil Aviation Administration of Korea N/A
South Korea (ROK)	Korea Office of Civil Aviation www.koca.go.kr

ASIA – PACIFIC

Australia	Civil Aviation Safety Authority www.casa.gov.au
Cook Islands	Pacific Aviation Safety Office www.paso.aero

Fiji	Civil Aviation Authority of Fiji www.caafi.org.fj
Kiribati	Pacific Aviation Safety Office www.paso.aero
Marshall Islands	Directorate of Civil Aviation of the Marshall Islands www.rmipa.com/airports/
Nauru	Pacific Aviation Safety Office www.paso.aero
New Zealand	Civil Aviation Authority of New Zealand www.caa.govt.nz
Niue	Pacific Aviation Safety Office www.paso.aero
Papua New Guinea	Civil Aviation Safety Authority of Papua New Guinea www.casapng.gov.pg
Philippines	Civil Aviation Authority of the Philippines www.caap.gov.ph
Samoa	Pacific Aviation Safety Office www.paso.aero
Solomon Islands	Pacific Aviation Safety Office www.paso.aero
Tonga	Pacific Aviation Safety Office www.paso.aero
Tuvalu	Pacific Aviation Safety Office www.paso.aero
Vanuatu	Pacific Aviation Safety Office www.paso.aero

ASIA – CENTRAL

Afghanistan	Ministry of Transport and Civil Aviation www.motca.gov.af
Armenia	General Department of Civil Aviation of Armenia www.aviation.am
Azerbaijan	State Civil Aviation Administration of Azerbaijan www.caa.gov.az
Georgia	Georgian Civil Aviation Agency www.gcaa.ge
Kazakhstan	Civil Aviation Committee www.aviation.mid.gov.kz
Kyrgyzstan	Civil Aviation Agency of Kyrgyz Republic (Kyrgyzstan) www.caa.kg
Tajikistan	Ministry of Transport - Civil Aviation Dept www.mintrans.tj/en
Turkmenistan	National Civil Aviation Authority Tel: +993 12-351-052
Uzbekistan	Civil Aviation Administration of Uzbekistan www.uzcaa.uz

ASIA – SOUTH

Bangladesh	Civil Aviation Authority, Bangladesh www.caab.gov.bd
Bhutan	Department of Civil Aviation of Bhutan www.dca.gov.bt
India	Directorate General of Civil Aviation www.dgca.nic.in
Maldives	Civil Aviation Department of the Maldives www.aviainfo.gov.mv

Nepal	Civil Aviation Authority of Nepal www.caanepal.org.np
Pakistan	Pakistan Civil Aviation Authority www.caapakistan.com.pk
Sri Lanka	Civil Aviation Authority of Sri Lanka www.caa.lk

ASIA – SE

Brunei	Department of Civil Aviation of Brunei www.civil-aviation.gov.bn
Cambodia	Secretariat of State for Civil Aviation www.civilaviation.gov.kh
Indonesia	Directorate General of Civil Aviation www.hubud.dephub.go.id
Laos	Department of Civil Aviation of Laos Tel: +856 21-512164
Macau	Civil Aviation Authority www.aacm.gov.mo
Malaysia	Department of Civil Aviation of Malaysia www.dca.gov.my
Myanmar	Department of Civil Aviation of Myanmar www.mot.gov.mm
Singapore	Civil Aviation Authority of Singapore www.caas.gov.sg
Taiwan	Civil Aeronautics Administration www.caa.gov.tw
Thailand	The Civil Aviation Authority of Thailand www.caat.or.th

Timor-Leste	Civil Aviation Division of Timor-Leste www.gov.east-timor.org/CAA/
Vietnam	Civil Aviation Administration of Vietnam www.caa.gov.vn

EUROPE

EU - EASA	European Aviation Safety Agency www.easa.europa.eu
Albania	Albanian Civil Aviation Authority www.aac.gov.al
Austria	Federal Ministry for Transport, Innovation & Technology www.bmvit.gv.at
Belgium	Federal Public Service Mobility and Transport www.mobilit.fgov.be/fr/
Bosnia and Herzegovina	Bosnia and Herzegovina Directorate of Civil Aviation www.bhdca.gov.ba
Bulgaria	Directorate General Civil Aviation Administration www.caa.bg
Croatia	Croatian Civil Aviation Agency www.ccaa.hr
Cyprus	Department of Civil Aviation of Cyprus www.mcw.gov.cy
Czech Republic	Civil Aviation Authority of the Czech Republic www.caa.cz
Denmark	Danish Transport Authority www.trafikstyrelsen.dk
Estonia	Estonian Civil Aviation Administration www.ecaa.ee

Finland	Finnish Transport Safety Agency www.trafi.fi
France	Directorate General for Civil Aviation www.dgac.fr
Germany	Federal Office for Civil Aviation of Germany www.lba.de/EN/
Greece	Hellenic Civil Aviation Authority www.hcaa.gr
Iceland	Icelandic Transport Authority www.icetra.is
Ireland	Irish Aviation Authority www.iaa.ie
Isle of Man	Isle of Man Aircraft Registry www.gov.im/ded/aircraft/
Italy	Italian Civil Aviation Authority www.enac-italia.it
Kosovo	Civil Aviation Authority of Kosovo www.caa-ks.org
Latvia	Civil Aviation Agency of Latvia www.caa.lv
Liechtenstein	Office of Civil Aviation of Liechtenstein www.bazl.admin.ch
Lithuania	Civil Aviation Administration of Lithuania www.caa.lt
Luxembourg	Directorate of Civil Aviation of Luxembourg www.dac.public.lu
Macedonia	Civil Aviation Agency of Macedonia www.dgca.gov.mk

Civilian Aviation Administrations by Region & Country

Malta	Civil Aviation Directorate of Malta www.transport.gov.mt/aviation/civil-aviation-directorate
Monaco	Monaco Civil Aviation Authority www.en.gouv.mc/Civil-Aviation-Authority
Montenegro	Civil Aviation Agency of Montenegro www.caa.me
Netherlands	Human Environment and Transport Inspectorate www.ilent.nl/onderwerpen/transport/luchtvaart/
Norway	Civil Aviation Authority of Norway www.luftfartstilsynet.no/caa_no/
Poland	Civil Aviation Office www.ulc.gov.pl
Portugal	National Institute of Civil Aviation of Portugal www.anac.pt
Romania	Romanian Civil Aeronautical Authority www.caa.ro
San Marino	San Marino Civil Aviation and Maritime Authority www.caa-mna.sm
Serbia	Civil Aviation Directorate of Serbia www.cad.gov.rs
Slovakia	Civil Aviation Authority of the Slovak Republic www.caa.sk
Slovenia	Civil Aviation Directorate of Slovenia www.mzp.gov.si
Spain	General Directorate of Civil Aviation of Spain www.fomento.es
Sweden	Swedish Transport Agency www.transportstyrelsen.se

Switzerland		Federal Office of Civil Aviation www.bazl.admin.ch
United Kingdom		Civil Aviation Authority www.caa.co.uk

EURASIA

Belarus		Aviation Department of Belarus www.avia.by
Moldova		Civil Aviation Administration of Moldova www.en.caa.md
Russia		Federal Air Transport Agency www.favt.ru
Turkey		Directorate General of Civil Aviation of Turkey www.shgm.gov.tr
Ukraine		State Aviation Administration of Ukraine www.avia.gov.ua

MIDDLE EAST

Bahrain		Department of Civil Aviation Affairs www.caa.gov.bh
Iran		Civil Aviation Organisation of Iran www.cao.ir
Iraq		Directorate General of Civil Aviation of Iraq www.iraqcaa.com
Israel		Civil Aviation Authority www.caa.gov.il
Jordan		Civil Aviation Regulatory Commission of Jordan www.carc.jo
Kuwait		Directorate General of Civil Aviation www.dgca.gov.kw

Lebanon	Lebanese Civil Aviation Authority www.dgca.gov.lb
Oman	Directorate General of Civil Aviation and Meteorology www.paca.gov.om
Qatar	Civil Aviation Authority of Qatar www.caa.gov.qa
Syria	Syrian Civil Aviation Authority www.scaa.sy
United Arab Emirates	General Civil Aviation Authority www.gcaa.ae
Yemen	Civil Aviation and Meteorological Authority of Yemen www.cama.gov.ye

NORTH AMERICA

Canada	Transport Canada Civil Aviation Directorate www.tc.gc.ca/eng/civilaviation/menu.htm
Mexico	Directorate General of Civil Aviation of Mexico **www.sct.gob.mx/transporte-y-medicina preventiva/aeronautica-civil/inicio**
United States	Federal Aviation Administration www.faa.gov

NORTH AMERICA – CARRIBEAN

Aruba	Department of Civil Aviation of Aruba www.dca.gov.aw
Bahamas	Department of Civil Aviation of Bahamas www.bahamas.gov.bs
Barbados	Civil Aviation Department of Barbados www.bcad.gov.bb

Bermuda	Bermuda Department of Civil Aviation www.dca.gov.bm
Cayman Islands	Civil Aviation Authority of the Cayman Islands www.caacayman.com
Cuba	Institute of Civil Aeronautics of Cuba www.cubagob.cu
Dominican Republic	Dominican Institute of Civil Aviation www.idac.gov.do
Grenada	Eastern Caribbean Civil Aviation Authority (ECCAA) www.eccaa.aero
Haiti	Office of Civil Aviation www.eccaa.aero/
Jamaica	Jamaica Civil Aviation Authority www.jcaa.gov.jm
Trinidad and Tobago	Trinidad and Tobago Civil Aviation Authority www.caa.gov.tt
Turks and Caicos Islands	Turks and Caicos Islands Civil Aviation Authority www.tcicaa.org

CENTRAL AMERICA

Belize	Beliz Department of Civil Aviation www.civilaviation.gov.bz
Costa Rica	Directorate General of Civil Aviation of Costa Rica www.dgac.go.cr
El Salvador	Civil Aviation Authority of El Salvador www.aac.gob.sv
Guatemala	Directorate General of Civil Aviation of Guatemala www.dgacguate.com

Honduras	Dirección General de Aeronáutica Civil (DGAC) www.ahac.gob.hn
Nicaragua	Nicaraguan Institute of Civil Aviation www.inac.gob.ni
Panama	Civil Aviation Authority of Panama www.aeronautica.gob.pa

SOUTH AMERICA

Argentina	National Civil Aviation Administration www.anac.gov.ar
Bolivia	General Directorate of Civil Aviation of Bolivia www.dgac.gob.bo
Brazil	National Civil Aviation Agency of Brazil www.anac.gov.br
Chile	Directorate General of Civil Aviation www.dgac.gob.cl
Colombia	Special Administrative Unit of Civil Aeronautics www.aerocivil.gov.co
Ecuador	Directorate General of Civil Aviation of Ecuador www.aviacioncivil.gob.ec
French Guiana	Department of Civil Aviation (France) Tel.:+594 359 300
Guyana	Guyana Civil Aviation Authority www.gcaa-gy.org
Paraguay	National Directorate of Civil Aviation of Paraguay www.dinac.gov.py
Peru	Directorate General of Civil Aviation of Peru www.mtc.gob.pe

Suriname	Civil Aviation Department of Suriname www.cadsur.sr
Uruguay	Dirección Nacional de Aviatión Civil e Infreastructura Aeronáutica (DINACIA) www.dinacia.gub.uy
Venezuela	National Institute of Civil Aviation of Venezuela www.inac.gov.ve www.inac.gov.v

APPENDIX B

A Quantiative Approach: the Precede-Proceed Logic Model

The PRECEDE-PROCEED logic model [1,2] provides a framework for the formal assessment of need and the development of an organized plan to address the identified need. The tool can be used to organize the plan and optimize the efficiency of creating an air medical program or improving an existing program. The specific requirements identified in the models various phases will serve as the focal point for program creation and ongoing improvement. The subsequent data collection and analysis will allow for the creation of a project map and action plan. By identifying the necessary discrete variables that influence the practicality and sustainability of the program allows the leadership to focus their development efforts efficiently and effectively.

It is important that the mapping process and action plan possess three characteristics [1,2]:

- Fluidity: the steps in the planning process are sequential and build upon one another.
- Flexibility: the plan accounts for the needs of stakeholders and conditions that influence the proposed solution in ways that allow it to adjust to meet as many requirements as possible.
- Functionality: the plan results in an air medical program that solves the problem it was intended to solve.

Addressing healthcare system needs requires the consideration of a multitude of factors and interrelated elements. Solutions to complex problems need not be complex themselves. Applying the method results in a highly organized data set and associated analysis which lends clarity to the development of an air medical program.

PRECEDE

The first component of the model is called PRECEDE which is an acronym for Predisposing, Reinforcing, and Enabling constructs in Ecological Diagnosis and Evaluation. This component captures all of the necessary objective and subjective elements in the existing healthcare delivery system and relates them to the requirements an air medical program will address. The first five sections organize the data collection and analysis according to discrete categories. As with any complex system, each factor interacts with each other factor. The Precede component allows identification of the myriad elements and the interactions between them.

Phase 1. The Social Assessment:
Phase 2. The Epidemiological Assessment

Phase 3. The Behavioral and Environmental Assessment
Phase 4. The Ecological Assessment
Phase 5. The Administrative and Policy Assessment

Clarity comes from seeing the discreet elements individually and as they relate to each other and the whole. The linear organization of data and analysis helps identify what needs to occur before, during, and after in the planning process. Ultimately, the PRECEDE model helps organize data, and then analyzes and facilitates the creation of goals, action items, timelines, and budgets. When carried out correctly, each step of the process can be attempted in order, according to rank of importance and timing in the process.

PROCEED

The second component of the logic model is called PROCEED. This component includes the entire implementation and ongoing assessments of the air medical program. The last 4 phases organize the actions necessary to evaluate the impact of the air medical program and provides a framework to assess the impact of the program and ways it can be improved.

Phase 6. Implementation
Phase 7. Process Evaluation
Phase 8. Impact Evaluation
Phase 9. Outcome Evaluation

The model is comprised of nine phases, or steps.

The diagram below serves as a visual representation of the cognitive process. The model flows from right to left along the top of the diagram for the PRECEDE component and from left to right along the bottom of the diagram for the PROCEED component of the workflow map.

The first five phases in the PRECEDE component involve considerable data collection and analysis and represent the entire body of information relevant to the creation of an air medical program. The accumulated analysis can then be used to guide all subsequent decisions related to the function of the program. While the logic model presents a linear process with discrete variables organized in orderly fashion the actual process will be dynamic. The implementation of the air medical program will require careful attention to timing, allocation of resources, and coordination of activities.

A Quantiative Approach: the Precede-Proceed Logic Model

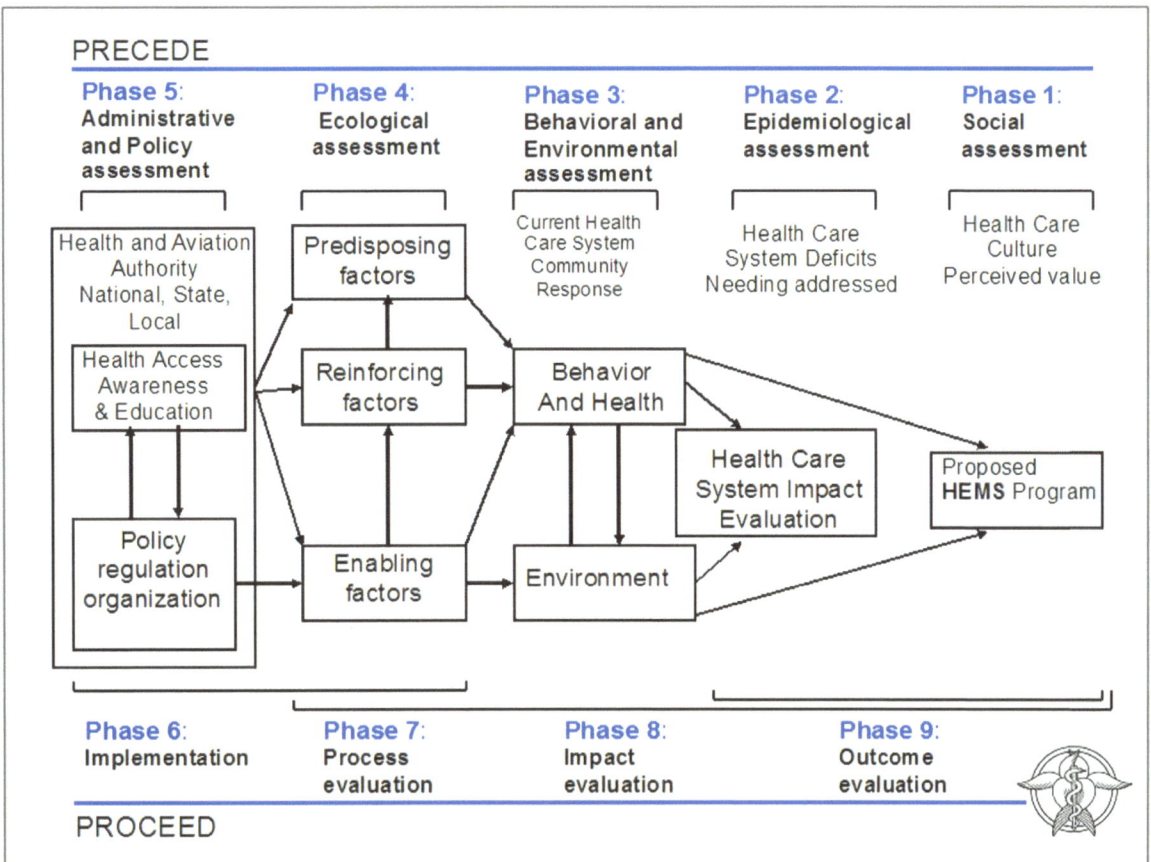

DETAILS OF THE PRECEDE METHODOLOGY

Phase 1: The Social Assessment

The social assessment analyzes the social variables that will support and/or confound the development of the air medical program. Stated another way, Phase 1 asks the user to examine all of the reasons why an air medical program has not existed previously and what attitudes and conditions they may encounter in setting up a new program. Users assess the attitudes, regulatory conditions, financial and human resources, and preexisting attitudes and conditions amongst various stakeholders as they relate to the acceptance of an air medical program. Understanding these dynamics and how they influence the existing healthcare infrastructure will allow one to account for and address them at the correct stage of development.

Interrelated factors for Phase 1

It is necessary to determine a common goal for all stakeholders by determining the social factors at play. Identify key attitudes and the associated educational efforts that may be directed at informing the various groups to facilitate support for the development and use of the air medical program.

Examples of social assessments:

- Demonstrate the clinical value and economic basis for introducing an air medical program in terms of outcomes (enhanced survival, improved recovery, reduced costs, etc.)
- Assess the willingness of regulatory agencies to allocate insurance funds or create an approved system for recovery of funds from insurance to pay for mission costs.
- Assess the willingness of air safety regulators to permit the introduction of novel technology to maximize the use of airspace, air routes, and approach/landing procedures to permit safe operations.
- Assess the willingness of airport operators and owners to accommodate rotary-wing and fixed-wing aircraft operations; including round-the-clock operations.
- Assess the attitudes of healthcare officials regarding their willingness to support the creation of an air medical program.
- Assess the attitudes held by members of the community and local population where the aircraft will be based to accept the impact of noise and landing zone operations within their communities.
- Assess the political will amongst the legislators and government officials regarding the creation of a favorable rules and regulations allowing appropriate licensure of an air medical program.
- Assess the willingness of funding sources to allocate the funds necessary to support the program.
- Assess the willingness of regulatory agencies to create the necessary regulatory changes to allow air medical program formation and function.
- Assess the attitudes of healthcare officials and clinicians to make referrals for their patients to the air medical service.
- Assess the willingness of clinicians in receiving facilities to accept patients from outlying areas.
- Assess the willingness of leaders from existing healthcare institutions to adapt their facilities and physical structure to accommodate a helicopter landing zone.
- Assess the willingness of public safety officials to educate and train their personnel in the required practices necessary to integrate air medical services into the existing public safety community.
- Assess the prevailing attitudes of the general public about supporting and using an air medical service in their community.

Phase 2: The Epidemiological Assessment

The epidemiological assessment allows for delineation of the extent, distribution, and root causes of a health access deficit in a defined population and location. This phase allows one to assess the extent of need and determine the level of service required to meet this need. This phase facilitates the estimates of the volume (daily, monthly, annual numbers) of transports, a necessary consideration when deciding how many aircraft and medical teams to field. It also becomes useful when determining where to base aircraft. Various validated tools exist to assist in predicting utilization for air medical services.[1,2]

Examples of epidemiological assessments:

- Assess the incidence and geographical distribution of trauma, cardiac, neurological, surgical, pediatric, and obstetrical conditions that would benefit from the care provided by an air medical service.

- Assess current referral patterns for patients with various health care conditions typically transported to hospitals.
- Assess current referral patterns for patients who must be transferred to other facilities for specialized care and the current duration of transport between the referring and accepting facilities.
- Analyze health records to identify other potential patients who would benefit from transfer by air medical service. For instance, identify patients who would have been transferred had an air medical program been available for assistance.
- Assess the current state of requests for emergency medical services from existing emergency responders.
- Determine the potential number of ill/injured patients that could benefit from the availability of AMS and calls for service by emergency responders if an air medical program were available.
- Assess loyalty to any existing transport services among providers and patients.
- Assess patterns of adverse events which may have been mitigated or prevented had an air medical service been available

Phase 3: Behavioral Assessment & Environmental Assessment

The behavioral assessment delineates the specific actions that will affect the implementation of the air medical program. This phase determines the current group behaviors including systems and processes that already exist as it relates to air medical services and the specific benefits a program would deliver.

The environmental assessment systematically assesses factors in the social and physical environment and their interaction or influence on a proposed air medical program.

Examples of behavioral factors:

- Current utilization patterns of critical care services present in the existing healthcare system
- Types and number of medical providers involved in providing critical care services both in hospital and out of hospital systems
- Current referral patterns between outlying providers and receiving facilities
- Current strategies used by local medical providers to make medical referrals to higher level centers
- Current use of air medical services among the population
- Potential for competition with existing medical transport services
- Potential for borders and territorial issues affecting response times of an air medical service

Examples of environmental factors:

- Description of existing healthcare infrastructure
- Emergency Dispatch capability (911 or other emergency phone numbers)
- Distance between patients with medical needs and the providers and facilities capable of treating them
- Distance between patients and the referring and receiving healthcare providers and centers

- Improved and unimproved roads
- Difficult terrain
- Territorial matters – border issues, territorial control, territorial disputes
- Political boundaries
- Weather patterns – prevalence of conditions which prevent safe flight (e.g., icing, fog, etc.)
- Concerns related to out-of-hospital time and its effects on the stability of the patient's clinical condition

Phase 4: Educational Assessment

The educational assessment delineates factors that predispose, enable, and reinforce a specific set of conditions or behaviors.

- Predisposing factors are any characteristics of a person or population that motivates behavior prior to the occurrence of the behavior,
- Enabling factors represent any characteristics of the environment that facilitates action and any skill or resource required to attain a specific behavior.
- Reinforcing factors are those that can be understood as incentives or disincentives following or perceived as a consequence of a behavior, either strengthening the affinity for or against the behavior.

The educational assessment phase identifies the prior experience, expectations, current attitudes, and beliefs related to air medical services amongst various stakeholders, the community, and any potential users. Information gathered in this phase will assist in creating educational programs to build support for the program. Additional efforts to educate the public, public safety officials, and healthcare leaders regarding air medical services will be required once the program begins delivering service.

At the same time, it is imperative to understand and mitigate the effect of negative attitudes regarding air medical services and the inconvenience of modifying current processes. Communicating with the various stakeholders, sharing the benefits and developing strategies to mitigate any negative impact (noise, expense, landing zone, policies and procedures at referring and receiving institutions, costs associated with helipad construction) will encourage discussion and facilitate acceptance. Ongoing communication with stakeholders and users will allow for active management of any conflicts and issues as they arise.

Successful air medical programs interact regularly with their stakeholders, partners, users, and prospective users through ongoing dialogue and educational offerings. Constant contact with all invested parties allows the service to inform them of their activities and stay abreast of any changes affecting the use and usefulness of the service. Stakeholders and prospective users will accept, support and utilize an air medical program if they remain confident that the service improves access to care, represents a safe and expedient alternative to current options, and meets the social and economic needs of the community. Long term success comes through excellent service and constant interaction with these groups to assure the service continually meets the identified need. Anticipating the concerns of supporters and detractors will assist in developing a communication strategy that will encourage acceptance while allaying concerns regarding the impact of the program on the healthcare system and the people it serves.

Examples of education assessments:

- Assess the current level of awareness of the benefits of air medical services amongst the healthcare system, its leadership, clinicians, and administrators.
- Assess the current level of awareness of air medical services amongst the general population.
- Assess the current level of preparation for interacting with medical helicopters amongst the public safety agencies in the community
- Determine any gaps in training amongst first responders and emergency dispatchers regarding the appropriate use of an air medical service for primary response service.

Examples of Educational Initiatives to enhance awareness of air medical services.

Pre-design phase

Develop and present white papers and other informative documents to legislators, potential supporters, and potential funding partners to initiate discussions and answer questions. These efforts will clarify the need and help build support for the creation of a new air medical program.

Design phase

Educational meetings and other forms of consensus building amongst key stakeholders, health care system leadership, and aviation authorities will assist the developers in fine tuning the design of the program and its key service offerings.

Implementation phase

Many methods exist for informing the public and healthcare workers about air medical services. Excellent programs maintain an active outreach and communication programs through a variety of media outlets and educational offerings. It will be helpful to begin educating the public and potential users about the purpose and capability of the air medical program prior to the first day of service. Ideally, the healthcare system will be prepared to use the service on the first day of operations. It is best to prepare in advance by providing key personnel with the knowledge and information they need to request support. This always includes a description of who should be referred for air medical services and how the service can be reached for referral.

Special attention must be given to educating referring institutions in the best way to interact with the helicopter and medical team. Air medical services involve complex patient movements outside the hospital. Many providers and facilities will be unfamiliar with coordinating a transfer by helicopter if they have never had access to air medical services.

The general public represents the largest pool of potential users. Ongoing outreach via public safety messages and public relations events allow the population to gain familiarity with the service and learn about the benefits of supporting air medical services. This becomes increasing important as programs seek funding from public sources and charitable donations. Maintaining a continuous positive presence in the public eye will greatly enhance acceptance and ongoing support for the program.

Ongoing Educational Initiatives

In addition to air medical operations training, many successful programs also offer ongoing educational programs for clinicians, emergency responders, safety personnel, in the form of continuing medical education programs, landing zone training classes, and ride-along programs.

- Sponsored Continuing Medical and Nursing Education Courses
- Site visits to educate referring clinicians in the benefits of your service
- Landing Zone Training- referring facilities, emergency responder services, fire and police
- Emergency Responder Training
- Joint Training opportunities with law enforcement, military and other public safety forces
- Ride along programs
- Medical Provider training and education
- Certificate programs in flight medicine and air medical services for staff recruitment and retention

Phase 5: Administrative Assessment

The administrative assessment takes into account all of the policies, necessary legal resources, stakeholder interactions, and surrounding circumstances prevailing in an organization (formal or informal) or regulatory body to facilitate or hinder the development of the air medical program.

Examples of administrative assessments:

- Regulations concerning licensing of air medical services
- Regulations affecting aviation operations in urban areas
- Regulations affecting helicopter aviation landing zone operations
- Laws and regulations affecting the scope of practice of medical providers working in AMS
- National, regional, and local laws and bylaws affecting the practice of medicine
- Reimbursement policies and procedures for covering the costs of air medical transport

Resources for many of the policies and procedures necessary for optimal program functioning exist online as free publications, online protocols, and as part of the accreditation process.

ORGANIZING THE DATA GATHERED IN PHASES 1-5

As noted in the logic model diagram, the first five phases represent categories of data relevant to the creation of an air medical program. Significant overlap exists between the various phases and in many cases data elements in one phase will interact with data in another phase. Noting these overlapping elements and analyzing the interplay between them will develop valuable insights into potential opportunities to positively attend to the issue while also avoiding oversights that may lead to delays in implementation.

We recommend assembling a series of data sets organized around the first five phases, with specific elements placed into their correct categories. It may also prove helpful to note along with each element the other interacting elements. Having visibility over all of the various elements will provide the opportunity to manage the elements successfully.

Analyzing the Data and Creating the Workflow Map

Once the users have identified the elements within the first five phases of the Precede component, they can begin to make determinations of the influence those factors will have on the program. They can begin to develop strategies to create an air medical service profile that meets as many needs as possible. The analysis will help in defining specific steps that must be taken to achieve the goal of creating a useful service that meets the identified needs.

Users can begin to assemble the necessary action steps into a work plan. Each step will have an ideal timing and completion time. Many steps interact with other steps, it is useful to view these interactions in advance and plan for the possibility of opportunities to accomplish several tasks at the same time and anticipate delays due to conflicts between competing steps.

Assessing the program's impact on the community and its integration into the healthcare system requires ongoing assessments. Interacting with stakeholders and patients after providing service allows the program to evaluate its performance and make improvements when necessary. Monitoring the changes in the healthcare system and the integration of air medical services allows the program to adapt to the evolving needs of the community. This process of building the program and measuring the ongoing workflow transfers directly into the maintanence of the program and adapting to changes in the healthcare system.

STAGE 2 - PROCEED: IMPLEMENTING THE AIR MEDICAL PROGRAM

The second component of the logic model, the PROCEED Stage, consists of four phases numbered six through nine. These phases represent the strategic implementation of the program based on what was learned from the assessments and analysis in phases 1 -5. They also include assessments of the processes put forward and whether the air medical program is meeting its goals and creating the intended outcomes.

Phase 6: Implementation:

Phase 6 requires the conversion of program objectives into actions including policy changes, regulatory adjustments, creation of the teams, educational programs and finally building out the complete air medical program.

Phase 7: Program Evaluation (Looking Inward At The Program)

Phase 7 requires the user to assess policies, materials, personnel, performance, quality of practice and services. Simply stated "Do the personnel, systems, and processes they use create the function and service profile we intend in order to meet the objectives we stated?"

Examples of program evaluation:

- Are we transporting the patients who need to be transported?
- Does our recruiting program assist us in reaching the most qualified staff?
- Does our flight maintenance program provide us with the aircraft availability and reliability we require?
- Does our reimbursement scheme meet the financial requirements of maintaining the program?

Phase 8: Impact Evaluation:

In this phase, the model looks outward at the program's interactions with the existing healthcare system. Phase 8 seeks to answer several questions about the program's external interactions.

Examples of impact evaluation:

- Is the air medical program creating the intended changes in access to critical care?
- Is the healthcare system adapting to integrate the air medical program into day to day operations?
- Assess program effects on intermediate objectives including changes in the predisposing, enabling, and reinforcing factors amongst behavioral and environmental changes?

Phase 9: Outcome Evaluation: DOES IT MAKE A MEANINGFUL DIFFERENCE

Phase 9 points to the need for recurring assessments of the effect the air medical program has on the lives of the people it serves and the outcome of their care. Studying the outcomes of an intervention allows planners to understand what is working, what is not working and how to further improve the system.

Examples of outcome evaluations:

- Are we improving survival and other relevant outcomes for the patients we serve?
- Does the program deliver a high level of clinical care to the intended population in an efficient and cost-effective manner?
- Do the various stakeholders benefit from the program to the intended extent?
- Has the program enhanced access to specialized care?

- Has the program reduced the time to definitive intervention?
- Has the program resulted in improving survival or return to work statistics for the affected populations?

This evaluation process allows leaders to determine which elements of the program are working correctly and helps identify areas that could be improved. Ideally, performing regular outcome evaluations allows for a continuous quality improvement process. Each assessment presents an opportunity for the program to adjust to changing needs and take advantage of new opportunities for expansion and improvements.

REFERENCES

Chapter 1 References

1. McGinnis KK. Rural and frontier EMS agenda for the future. National Rural Health Association. 2004. Available at: www.nrharural.org. Accessed 2005, December 20.

2. Foundation for Air Medical Research and Education. Air medicine: Accessing the Future of Health Care, Alexandria, Virginia, 2006.

3. Julinek T. Opening remarks, Minister of Health for the Czech Republic, AirMed 2008, Prague, Czech Republic, May 2008.

4. Macione AR, Wilcox DE. Utilization prediction for helicopter services. Ann Emerg Med 1997; 16(4):391-398.

5. World Health Organization (2009). Global Forum on Trauma Care: Meeting Report. Retrieved from: http://www.who.int/emergencycare/trauma/global_forum_meeting_report.pdf

6. Press GM, Miller SK, Hassan IA, Alade KH, Camp E, Junco DD, Holcomb JB. Prospective evaluation of prehospital trauma ultrasound during aeromedical transport. J Emerg Med. 2014 Dec; 47(6):638-45.

7. Kashyap R, Anderson P, Vakil A, Russi CS, Cartin-Ceba R. A retrospective comparison of helicopter transport versus ground transport in patients with severe sepsis and septic shock. Int J Emerg Med. 2016 Dec;9(1):15.

8. Hutton CF, Fleming J, Youngquist S, Hutton KC, Heiser DM, Barton ED. Stroke and Helicopter Emergency Medical Service Transports: An Analysis of 25,332 Patients. Air Med J. 2015 Nov-Dec;34(6):348-56.

9. Jones R, Langford S. Australia's flying doctors. How the world's largest aeromedical response service provides effective patient retrieval in the Outback. JEMS. 2015 Apr; 40(4):39-43.

10. Østerås Ø, Brattebø G, Heltne J K. Helicopter-based emergency medical services for a sparsely populated region: A study of 42,500 dispatches. Acta Anaesthesiol Scand. 2016 May; 60(5):659-67.

11. Concannon TW et al, Comparative effectiveness of ST segment–elevation myocardial infarction regionalization strategies. Circulation: Cardiovasc Qual Outcomes. September 2010; 3:506-513.

12. Bruhn JD, Williams KA, Aghababian R. True costs of air medical vs. ground ambulance systems. Air Med J1993; 12(8):262-268.

13. Gearhart PA, et al. Cost-effectiveness analysis of helicopter EMS for trauma patients. Ann Emerg Med 1997; 30(4); 500-506.

14. Teng TO. Five hundred life-saving interventions and their cost effectiveness. Society for Risk Analysis. 1995; 15:3.

15. Giannakopoulos GF, Kolodzinskyi MN, Christiaans HM, Boer C, de Lange-de Klerk ES, Zuidema WP, Bloemers FW, Bakker FC. Helicopter Emergency Medical Services save lives: outcome in a cohort of 1073 polytraumatized patients. Eur J Emerg Med. 2013 Apr; 20(2):79-85.

16. Brown JB, Leeper CM, Sperry JL, Peitzman AB, Billiar TR, Gaines BA, Gestring ML. Helicopters and injured kids: Improved survival with scene air medical transport in the pediatric trauma population. J Trauma Acute Care Surg. 2016 May; 80(5):702-10.

17. Andruszkow H, Hildebrand F, Lefering R, Pape HC, Hoffmann R, Schweigkofler U. Ten years of helicopter emergency medical services in Germany: do we still need the helicopter rescue in multiple traumatized patients? Injury. 2014 Oct; 45 Supplement 3:S53-8.

18. Levick NR, Emergency Medical Services: Unique Transportation Safety Challenge, Report No. 08-3010, Transportation Research Board, January 2008 Page 3. Accessed 2011, March. Retrieved from: http://www.objectivesafety.net/LevickTRB08-3010CD.pdf

19. Blumen IJ et al. A safety review and risk assessment in air medical transport. Supplement to the Air Medical Physicians Handbook. Air Medical Physicians Association 2002; 2-67.

20. Zalstein S1, Cameron PA. Helicopter emergency medical services: their role in integrated trauma care. Aust N Z J Surg. 1997 Sep; 67(9):593-8.

21. Baxt WG, Moody P. The impact of rotorcraft aeromedical emergency care service on trauma mortality. JAMA 1983; 249:3047-51.

22. Baxt WG, et al. Hospital-based rotorcraft aeromedical emergency care services and trauma mortality: a multicenter study. Ann Emerg Med 1985; 14:859-64.

23. Baxt WG, Moody P. The impact of advanced prehospital emergency care on the mortality of severely brain-injured patients. J Trauma 1987; 27:365-9.

24. Topol EJ, Fung AY, Kline E, et al. Safety of helicopter transport and out-of-hospital intravenous fibrinolytic therapy in patients with evolving myocardial infarction. Catheter Cardiovasc Diagn 1986; 12:151-5.

25. Grines CL, et al. A randomized trial of transfer for coronary angioplasty versus on-site thrombolysis in patients with high-risk myocardial infarction. J Am Coll Cardiol 2002; 39:1713-9(3-11).

26. Kaplan L, et al. Emergency aeromedical transport of patients with acute myocardial infarction. Ann Emerg Med 1987; 16:55-7.

27. Tyson AA, et al. Plasma catecholamine levels in patients transported by helicopter for acute myocardial infarction and unstable angina pectoris. Am J Emerg Med 1988; 6:435-8.

28. Rodgers G, et al. Helicopter transport of patients with acute myocardial infarction. Tex Med. 1988; 84:35-7.

29. Gore JM, et al. Feasibility and safety of emergency interhospital transport of patients during early hours of acute myocardial infarction. Arch Intern Med 1989; 149:353-5.

30. Vukov LF, Johnson DQ. External transcutaneous pacemakers in interhospital transport of cardiac patients. Ann Emerg Med 1989; 18:738-40.

31. Fromm RE, et al. Bleeding complications following initiation of thrombolytics therapy for acute myocardial infarction: a comparison of helicopter-transported and non-transported patients. Ann Emerg Med 1991; 20:892-5.

32. Thomas SH, Harrison T, Wedel SK, Thomas DP. Helicopter emergency medical services roles in disaster operations. Prehosp Emerg Care. 2000 Oct-Dec; 4(4):338-44.

Chapter 3 References

Green LW, Kreuter MW. Health Program Planning: An Educational and Ecological Approach. 4th edition. New York, NY, USA: McGraw-Hill Higher Education; 2005.

Crosby R1, Noar SM. What is a planning model? An introduction to PRECEDE-PROCEED. J Public Health Dent. 2011 Winter; 71 Supplement 1: S7-15.

Chapter 4 References

1. Marinangeli F, Tomei M, Ursini ML, Ricotti V, Varrassi G. Helicopter emergency medical service in Italy: reality and perspectives. Air Med J. 2007 Nov-Dec; 26(6):292-8.

2. Doctor on board? What is the optimal skill-mix in military pre-hospital care? Emerg Med J 2011; 28:882 – 883)

3. Wirtz, MH; Cayten, CG, et al (Paramedic Versus Nurse Crews in the Helicopter Transport of Trauma Patients, Air Medical Journal January – February 2002).

4. Putzke M1. [Medical doctor in mountain rescue service - a profession's perspective]. [Article in German]. Anasthesiol Intensivmed Notfallmed Schmerzther. 2008 Jan; 43(1):74-7

Chapter 6 References

1. International Helicopter Safety Team: Our Vision an International Community with Zero Accidents. Retrieved from: http://www.ihst.org/Default.aspx?tabid=3043&language=en-US

2. The Association of Air Medical Services. Vision Zero= Education. Awareness. Vigilance. Retrieved from: http://aams.org/vision-zero/

3. The Association of Air Medical Services. Safety Management Training Academy. Retrieved from: http://aams.org/events/smta/

4. Flight Safety. A Roadmap to a Just Culture: Enhancing the Safety Environment. Retrieved from: http://flightsafety.org/files/just_culture.pdf

Chapter 7 References

1. CareFlight is Now Life Flight. Retrieved from: https://www.careflight.org.au/page/what-we-do/

Chapter 8 References

1. Schuurman N1, Bell NJ, L'Heureux R, Hameed SM. Modelling optimal location for pre-hospital helicopter emergency medical services. BMC Emerg Med. 2009 May 9;9:6.

2. Røislien J, van den Berg PL, Lindner T, Zakariassen E, Aardal K, van Essen JT. Exploring optimal air ambulance base locations in Norway using advanced mathematical modelling. Inj Prev. 2016 Jun 20.

3. McQueen C1, Crombie N2, Cormack S2, Wheaton S3. Medical Emergency Workload of a Regional UK HEMS Service. Air Med J. 2015 May-Jun; 34(3):144-8. doi: 10.1016/j.amj.2014.12.013.

4. Brown JB1, Gestring ML, Guyette FX, Rosengart MR, Stassen NA, Forsythe RM, Billiar TR, Peitzman AB, Sperry JL. Development and Validation of the Air Medical Prehospital Triage Score for Helicopter Transport of Trauma Patients. Ann Surg. 2015 Oct 22.

5. Stewart CL, Metzger RR, Pyle L, Darmofal J, Scaife E, Moulton SL. Helicopter versus ground emergency medical services for the transportation of traumatically injured children. J Pediatr Surg. 2015 Feb; 50(2):347-52.

6. Michailidou M, Goldstein SD, Salazar J, Aboagye J, Stewart D, Efron D, Abdullah F, Haut ER. Helicopter overtriage in pediatric trauma. J Pediatr Surg. 2014 Nov; 49(11):1673-7.

7. Stewart K, Garwe T, Bhandari N, Danford B, Albrecht R. Factors Associated with the Use of Helicopter Inter-facility Transport of Trauma Patients to Tertiary Trauma Centers within an Organized Rural Trauma System. Prehosp Emerg Care. 2016 Mar 17:1-10

8. Thomas DP, Thomas SH; I 2002-2003 Air Medical Services Committee of the NAEMSP. Guidelines for air medical dispatch. Prehosp. Emerg Care 2003; 7:265-271. Retrieved from: http://www.ebmedicine.net/topics.php?paction=showTopicSeg&topic_id=80&seg_id=1609

9. ACEP Policy Paper: GUIDELINES FOR AIR MEDICAL DISPATCH Policy Resource and Education Paper American College of Emergency Physicians and National Association of EMS Physicians Approved January 2006. Retrieved from: https://www.acep.org/uploadedFiles/ACEP/Practice_Resources/issues_by_category/Emergency_Medical_Services/GuidelinesForAirMedDisp.pdf

10. Matsumoto H. et al. Dispatch of Helicopter Emergency Medical Services via Advanced Automatic Collision Notification. J Emerg Med. 2016 Mar; 50(3):437-43.

Chapter 11 References

1. Wright SW, Lindsell CJ, Hinckley WR, Williams A, Holland C, Lewis CH, Heimburger G. High fidelity medical simulation in the difficult environment of a helicopter: feasibility, self-efficacy and cost. BMC Med Educ. 2006 Oct 5; 6:49.

2. Matics D. Implementing Simulation in Air Medical Training: Integration of Adult Learning Theory. Air Med J. 2015 Sep-Oct; 34(5):261-2.

3. Alfes CM, Steiner SL, Manacci CF. Critical Care Transport Training: New Strides in Simulating the Austere Environment. Air Med J. 2015 Jul-Aug; 34(4):186-7.

4. Bender GJ, Kennally K. Implementing a Neonatal Transport System with Simulation in Kosovo. Air Med J. 2016 May-Jun; 35(3):126-31. Retrieved from: www.bw-zsa.org/simulation